Acute and Critical Care Formulas and Laboratory Values

AF167638

Acute and Critical Care Formulas and Laboratory Values

Joseph Varon, MD, FACP,
FCCP, FCCM

University of Texas Health Science Center,
Houston, TX, USA

Robert E. Fromm, Jr., MD, MPH, FACP,
FCCP, FCCM

University of Arizona College of Medicine,
Phoenix, AZ, USA

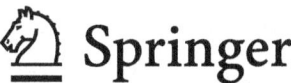 Springer

Joseph Varon, MD, FACP, FCCP,
    FCCM
Department of Critical Care
    Services
University General Hospital

Department of Acute and
    Continuing Care
The University of Texas Health
    Science Center
Houston, TX, USA

Robert E. Fromm, Jr., MD, MPH,
    FACP, FCCP, FCCM
Maricopa Integrated Health System
Department of Internal Medicine
University of Arizona College
    of Medicine
Phoenix, AZ, USA

ISBN 978-1-4614-7509-5   ISBN 978-1-4614-7510-1 (eBook)
DOI 10.1007/978-1-4614-7510-1
Springer New York Heidelberg Dordrecht London

Library of Congress Control Number: 2013945396

Printed on acid-free paper

Springer is part of Springer Science+Business Media (www.springer.com)

*We wish to dedicate this book to Robert E Fromm III.
A bright, kind, and gentle soul, who left us long
before his time. The straightforward approach
of this book and its clear, concise style are very
reminiscent of Rob. You are missed.*

Preface

The fields of *Acute* and *Critical Care Medicine* are relatively new. Over the past few decades, we have seen an enormous growth in the number of intensive care units (ICUs) and free standing Emergency Departments (EDs) in the USA. Thousands of medical students, residents, fellows, attending physicians, critical care nurses, pharmacists, respiratory therapists, and other healthcare providers (irrespective of their ultimate field of practice) spend several months or years of their professional lives, taking care of acutely ill or severely injured patients. Practitioners must be able to interpret clinical data obtained by many kinds of monitoring devices, apply formulas, understand laboratory values, and then integrate this information with their knowledge of the pathophysiology of disease.

This handbook is based on the first edition of the *ICU Handbook of Facts, Formulas, and Laboratory Values,* which we wrote more than a decade ago. The original handbook was written for everyone engaged in Critical Care Medicine. In this new book, we have attempted to present basic and generally accepted clinical formulas as well as laboratory values and tables, which we feel will be useful to the practitioner of Acute Care and Critical Care Medicine. In addition, formulas that help explain physiologic concepts or that underlie clinical measurements or diagnostic tests, even if not clinically useful themselves, are included. Multiple methods for deriving a particular quantity are included where appropriate. The formulas presented in the chapters of this book follow an outline format. The chapters are divided by organ system (i.e., neurologic disorders and cardiovascular disorders) as well as special topics (i.e., environmental disorders, trauma, and toxicology). A special chapter regarding laboratory values is provided. In addition, each chapter reviews some formulas systematically.

Acute and Critical Care Medicine are not static fields and changes occur every day. Therefore, this handbook is not meant to define the standard of care, but rather to be a general guide to current formulas and laboratory values used in the care of patients with Acute and Critical Care Medicine problems.

Houston, TX   **Joseph Varon, MD, FACP, FCCP, FCCM**
Phoenix, AZ   **Robert E. Fromm Jr., MD, MPH, FACP, FCCP, FCCM**

Acknowledgment

The authors wish to acknowledge the editorial assistance of Drs. Stephanie Pablo and German Tirado in the preparation of this book.

Contents

Preface   vii

1. Cardiovascular Facts and Formulas   1

2. Endocrinology and Metabolism Facts and Formulas   25

3. Environmental Facts and Formulas   33

4. Gastrointestinal Facts and Formulas   41

5. Hematological Facts and Formulas   45

6. Infectious Diseases Facts and Formulas   53

7. Neurological Facts and Formulas   57

8. Nutrition Facts and Formulas   71

9. Obstetrics and Gynecology Facts and Formulas   77

10. Oncology Facts and Formulas   83

11. Pediatric Facts, Formulas, and Laboratory Values   87

12. Pulmonary Facts and Formulas   101

13. Renal, Fluid, and Electrolyte Facts and Formulas   127

14. Statistics and Epidemiology: Facts and Formulas   141

15. Toxicology Facts and Formulas   149

16. Trauma Facts and Formulas   157

17. Common Laboratory Values   165

Key Telephone Numbers   173

Notes   175

Abbreviations   177

Index   187

1

Cardiovascular Facts and Formulas

The management of the critically ill patient requires considerable knowledge of cardiovascular performance, physiology, and the measurements of these parameters. Many therapies are aimed at altering one or more cardiovascular parameters, and, therefore, an understanding of the relation between these variables is essential.

The clinical assessment of cardiovascular performance has improved importantly over the past several decades. However, an ideal method of monitoring blood flow remains to be developed. Noninvasive technical difficulties have precluded their widespread adoption in the ICU and emergency departments (ED). Undoubtedly, further refinements and new developments will arise in the years to come. In the ED and the ICU, a number of cardiovascular guiding principles should be kept in mind.

■ 1. PRESSURE = FLOW × RESISTANCE

This is true in the airways as well as in the cardiovascular system. For example:

Mean arterial pressure = cardiac output × systemic vascular resistance

Mean pulmonary arterial pressure = cardiac output × pulmonary vascular resistance

The unmeasured resistance term is usually calculated by solving the equations:

$$\text{Systemic vascular resistance} = \frac{\text{mean arterial pressure}}{\text{cardiac output}}$$

J. Varon and R.E. Fromm Jr., *Acute and Critical Care Formulas and Laboratory Values*, DOI 10.1007/978-1-4614-7510-1_1, © Springer Science+Business Media New York 2014

■ 2. PRIMARY DETERMINANTS

The primary determinants of cardiovascular performance are:

Heart rate	Preload
Afterload	Contractility

■ 3. OTHER PRINCIPLES AND CONVERSION FACTORS

Fluid flow

$$\textbf{Fluid flow} = \frac{(\text{pressure difference})(\text{radius})^4}{8(\text{vessel length})(\text{fluid viscosity})}$$

Conversion to mmHg

$$\textbf{Pressure in mmHg} = \text{Pressure in cm } H_2O \, / \, 1.36$$

Laplace's law

$$\textbf{Wall tension} = \text{distending pressure} \times \frac{\text{vessel radius}}{\text{wall thickness}}$$

Ohm's law

$$\textbf{Current (I)} = \frac{\text{electromotive force } (E)}{\text{resistance } (R)}$$

Poiseuille's law

$$\mathbf{Q} = v\pi r^2$$

where

Q = rate of blood flow (mm/s)

πr^2 = cross-sectional area (cm^2)

v = velocity of blood flow

Vascular capacitance

$$\textbf{Vascular compliance (capacitance)} = \frac{\text{increase in volume}}{\text{increase in pressure}}$$

Vascular distensibility

$$\textbf{Vascular distensibility} = \frac{\text{increase in volume}}{\text{increase in pressure} \times \text{original volume}}$$

■ 4. DIRECT MEASUREMENTS OF THE HEART RATE

Direct measurements of the heart rate are relatively easy. Preload, afterload, and contractility are more difficult to assess clinically. In assessment of cardiovascular performance, the following hemodynamic measurements are commonly measured or calculated:

Arteriovenous oxygen content difference [avDO$_2$]: This is the difference between the arterial oxygen content (CaO$_2$) and the venous oxygen content (CvO$_2$).

Body surface area (BSA): Calculated from height and weight, it is generally used to index measured and derived values according to the size of the patient.

Cardiac index (CI): calculated as cardiac output/BSA, it is the prime determinant of hemodynamic function.

Left ventricular stroke work index (LVSWI): It is the product of the stroke index (SI) and [Mean arterial pressure (MAP) – pulmonary artery occlusion pressure (PAOP)], and a unit correction factor of 0.0136. The LVSWI measures the work of the left ventricle (LV) as it ejects into the aorta.

$$\textbf{LVSWI} = 0.0136 \times \text{SI}(\text{MAP} - \text{PAOP})$$

Mean arterial pressure (MAP): Estimated as one-third of pulse pressure plus the diastolic blood pressure.

Oxygen consumption (VO$_2$): Calculated as $C(a-v)O_2 \times CO \times 10$, it is the amount of oxygen extracted in mL/min by the tissue from the arterial blood.

Oxygen delivery (DO$_2$): Calculated as $(CaO_2) \times CO \times 10$, it is the total oxygen delivered by the cardiorespiratory systems.

Pulmonary vascular resistance index (PVRI): Calculated as (MAP – PAOP)/CI, it measures the resistance in the pulmonary vasculature.

Right ventricular stroke work index (RVSWI): It is the product of the SI and [mean pulmonary artery pressure (MPAP) – central venous pressure (CVP)], and a unit correction factor of 0.0136. It measures the work of the right ventricle as it ejects into the pulmonary artery.

Stroke index (SI): Calculated as CI/heart rate, it is the average volume of blood ejected by the ventricle with each beat.

Systemic vascular resistance index (SVRI): Calculated as (MAP – CVP)/CI, it is the customary measure of the resistance in the systemic circuit.

Venous admixture (Qva/Qt): Calculated as $(CcO_2 - CaO_2)/(CcO_2 - CvO_2)$, it represents the fraction of cardiac output not oxygenated in an idealized lung.

■ 5. CARDIAC OUTPUT FORMULAS

$$\textbf{Output of left ventricle} = \frac{O_2 \text{ consumption (mL / min)}}{[AO_2] - [VO_2]}$$

$$= \frac{250\text{mL / min}}{190\text{mL / L arterial blood} - 140 \text{ mL / L venous blood in pulmonary artery}}$$

$$= \frac{250\text{mL / min}}{50\text{mL / L}} = 5\text{L / min}$$

It may also be measured by thermodilution techniques:

$$\mathbf{Q} = \frac{V(T_b - T_i)K}{\int T_b(t)\mathrm{d}t}$$

where

Q = cardiac output
V = volume of injectate
T_b = blood temperature
T_i = injectate temperature
K = a constant including the density factor and catheter characteristics
$\int T_b(t)\mathrm{d}t$ = area under the blood–temperature–time curve

The same principle is applicable for the pulmonary blood flow:

$$\mathbf{Q} = \frac{B}{(Cv - Ca)}$$

where

Q = pulmonary blood flow
B = rate of loss of the indicator of alveolar gas
Cv = concentration of the indicator in the venous blood
Ca = concentration of the indicator in the arterial blood

$$\mathbf{Q} = \frac{VO_2}{(CaO_2 - CvO_2)}$$

where

Q = total pulmonary blood flow
VO_2 = oxygen uptake
CaO_2 = arterial oxygen concentration
CvO_2 = venous oxygen content equation

■ 6. OTHER CARDIOVASCULAR PERFORMANCE
FORMULAS/TABLES (SEE ALSO TABLES 1.1, 1.2,
AND 1.3)

Table 1.1 Normal hemodynamic parameters—adult

Parameter	Equation	Normal range
Arterial blood pressure (BP)	Systolic (SBP)	<120 mmHg
	Diastolic (DBP)	<80 mmHg
Mean arterial pressure (MAP)	$[SBP + (2 \times DBP)]/3$	70–105 mmHg
Right atrial pressure (RAP)		2–6 mmHg
Right ventricular pressure (RVP)	Systolic (RVSP)	15–25 mmHg
	Diastolic (RVDP)	0–8 mmHg
Pulmonary artery pressure (PAP)	Systolic (PASP)	15–25 mmHg
	Diastolic (PADP)	8–15 mmHg
Mean pulmonary artery pressure (MPAP)	$[PASP + (2 \times PADP)]/3$	10–20 mmHg
Pulmonary artery wedge pressure (PAWP)		6–12 mmHg
Left atrial pressure (LAP)		6–12 mmHg
Cardiac output (CO)	$HR \times SV/1,000$	4.0–8.0 L/min
Cardiac index (CI)	CO/BSA	2.5–4.0 L/min/m^2
Stroke volume (SV)	$CO/HR \times 1,000$	60–100 mL/beat
Stroke volume index (SVI)	$CI/HR \times 1,000$	33–47 mL/m^2/beat
Systemic vascular resistance (SVR)	$80 \times (MAP - RAP)/CO$	800–1,200 dyne•s/cm^5
Systemic vascular resistance index (SVRI)	$80 \times (MAP - RAP)/CI$	1,970–2,390 dyne•s/cm^5/m^2
Pulmonary vascular resistance (PVR)	$80 \times (MPAP - PAWP)/CO$	<250 dyne•s/cm^5
Pulmonary vascular resistance index (PVRI)	$80 \times (MPAP - PAWP)/CI$	255–285 dyne•s/cm^5/m^2

Table 1.2 Hemodynamic parameters—adult

Parameter	Equation	Normal range
Left ventricular stroke work (LVSW)	$SV \times (MAP - PAWP) \times 0.0136$	8–10 g/m/m^2
Left ventricular stroke work index (LVSWI)	$SVI \times (MAP - PAWP) \times 0.0136$	50–62 g/m^2/beat
Right ventricular stroke work (RVSW)	$SV \times (MPAP - RAP) \times 0.0136$	51–61 g/m/m^2
Right ventricular stroke work index (RVSWI)	$SV \times (MPAP - RAP) \times 0.0136$	5–10 g/m^2/beat
Coronary artery perfusion pressure (CPP)	Diastolic $(BP - PAWP)$	60–80 mmHg
Right ventricular end-diastolic volume (RVEDV)	SV/EF	100–160 mL
Right ventricular end-systolic volume (RVESV)	EDV–SV	50–100 mL
Right ventricular ejection fraction (RVEF)	SV/EDV	40–60 %

Alveolar – arterial O_2 difference or "A – a gradient" $=$ Alveolar pO_2 – arterial pO_2

Normal < 10 Torr

Alveolar pO_2 at sea level (PAO_2) $= (FIO_2 \times 713) - 1.2 \times PaCO_2$

Arterial blood O_2 content (CaO_2) $= (PaO_2 \times 0.003)$
$+ (1.34 \times Hb \text{ in gms} \times \text{arterial blood Hb } O_2 \text{ sat}\%)$

Normal $= 18$–20 mL/dL

Arteriovenous Oxygen difference $(avDO_2)$ $= (CaO_2) - (CvO_2)$

Normal $= 4$–5 mL/dL

Cardiac index (CI) $=$ cardiac output / body surface area

$Normal = 3.0 - 3.4 \text{L} / \min\text{m}^2$
$= \% \dfrac{\text{end-diastolic volume} - \text{end-systolic volume}}{\text{end-diastolic volume}}$

Table 1.3 Oxygenation parameters—adult

Parameter	Equation	Normal range
Partial pressure of arterial oxygen (PaO_2)		80–100 mmHg
Partial pressure of arterial CO_2 ($PaCO_2$)		35–45 mmHg
Bicarbonate (HCO_3)		22–26 mEq/L
pH		7.35–7.45
Arterial oxygen saturation (SaO_2)		95–100 %
Mixed venous saturation (SvO_2)		60–80 %
Arterial oxygen content (CaO_2)	$(0.0138 \times Hb \times SaO_2) + 0.0031 \times PaO_2$	16–22 mL/dL
Venous oxygen content (CvO_2)	$(0.0138 \times Hb \times SvO_2) + 0.0031 \times PvO_2$	12–15 mL/dL
A–V oxygen content $[C(a-v)O_2]$	$CaO_2 - CvO_2$	4–6 mL/dL
Oxygen delivery (DO_2)	$CaO_2 \times CO \times 10$	950–1,150 mL/dL
Oxygen delivery index (DO_2I)	$CaO_2 \times CI \times 10$	500–600 mL/min/m^2
Oxygen consumption (VO_2)	$[C(a-v)O_2] \times CO \times 10$	200–250 mL/min
Oxygen consumption index (VO_2I)	$[C(a-v)O_2] \times CI \times 10$	120–160 mL/min/m^2
Oxygen extraction ration (O_2ER)	$[(CaO_2 - CvO_2)/CaO_2] \times 100$	22–30 %
Oxygen extraction index (O_2EI)	$(SaO_2 - SvO_2)/SaO_2 \times 100$	20–25 %

Mean arterial (or pulmonary) pressure $= DBP + 1/3 (SBP - DBP)$

Mean pulmonary arterial pressure $= DPAP + 1/3 (SPAP - DPAP)$

O_2 delivery index (DO_2I) $= CaO_2 \times$ cardiac index $\times 10$

Normal $= 500$–600 mL/min-m^2

O$_2$ consumption index (VO$_2$I) = Arteriovenous O$_2$ difference × cardiac index × 10

Normal = 120–160 %

O$_2$ extraction (O$_2$Ext) = (Arteriovenous O$_2$ difference / arterial blood O$_2$ content) × 100

Normal = 20–30 %

Pulmonary vascular resistance index (PVRI) = 79.92 (Mean PAP – PAOP) / CI

Normal = 255–285 dyne•s/cm^5•m^2

$$\text{Shunt } \% = \left(\frac{Q_s}{Q_t} \right)$$

$$\mathbf{Q}_s / \mathbf{Q}_t (\%) = \frac{CcO_2 - CaO_2}{CcO_2 - CvO_2}$$

$$\mathbf{CcO_2} = \text{Hb in gm} \times 1.34 + (\text{Alveolar pO}_2 \times 0.003)$$

Normal < 10%   *Considerable disease* = 20 – 29% *Life threatening* > 30%

$$\textbf{Pulmonary to systemic flow ratio (QP} - \textbf{QS)} = \frac{\text{Sat}_{(Ao)} - \text{Sat}_{(MV)}}{\text{Sat}_{(PV)} - \text{Sat}_{(PA)}}$$

Sat$_{(Ao)}$ = saturation aorta (%)
Sat$_{(MV)}$ = saturation mixed venous (%)
Sat$_{(PV)}$ = saturation pulmonary venous (%)
Sat$_{(PA)}$ = saturation pulmonary artery (%)

It is useful in the evaluation of cardiac shunts

Stroke volume (SV) $= (\text{end} - \text{diastolic volume}) - (\text{end} - \text{systolic volume})$

Systemic vascular resistance index (SVRI) $= 79.92 \left(\dfrac{\text{MAP} - \text{CVP}}{\text{CI}} \right)$

Normal $= 1{,}970{-}2{,}390$ dyne•s/cm^5•m^2

Venous blood O_2 content (CvO$_2$) $= (\text{PvO}_2 \times 0.003)$
$+ (1.34 \times \text{Hb in gm} \times \text{venous blood Hb } O_2 \text{ sat\%})$

Normal $= 13{-}16$ mL/dL

Pulse pressure variation (ΔPP) $= \dfrac{\text{PP}_{max} - \text{PP}_{min}}{(\text{PP}_{max} + \text{PP}_{min})/2}$

$$\text{PP}_{max} = P_{\text{sysMAX}} - P_{\text{diaMAX}}$$

$$\text{PP}_{min} = P_{\text{sysMIN}} - P_{\text{diaMIN}}$$

A ΔPP value of 13 % differentiates responders to nonresponders (<13 %) to a fluid challenge.

Shock index $=$ Heart rate / systolic blood pressure

Values ≥ 0.8 are suggestive of any kind of shock.

■   7. PACEMAKER TABLE (TABLE 1.4)

Table 1.4 Pacemaker Classification

Letter position	I *Chamber paced*	II *Chamber sensed*	III *Modes of response*	IV *Programmable functions*	V *Special antitachyarrhythmia functions*
Letters used	V - ventricle A - atrium D - double	V - ventricle A - atrium D - double O - none	T - triggered I - inhibited D - double O - none R - reverse	P - programmable (rate and/or output) M -multiprogrammable C - communicating O - none	B - bursts N - normal rate competition S - scanning E - external

■ 8. ELECTROCARDIOGRAPHIC FORMULAS/TABLES

Rate calculation:

Each large square = 0.2 s; 5 large squares/s.

For specific rate, measure *R–R* interval as shown in Table 1.5.

Table 1.5 Heart rate determination in electrocardiogram by counting the *R–R* intervals

1	300 beat/min
2	150 bpm
3	100 bpm
4	75 bpm
5	60 bpm
6	50 bpm

Axis determination (see Figs. 1.1 and 1.2):

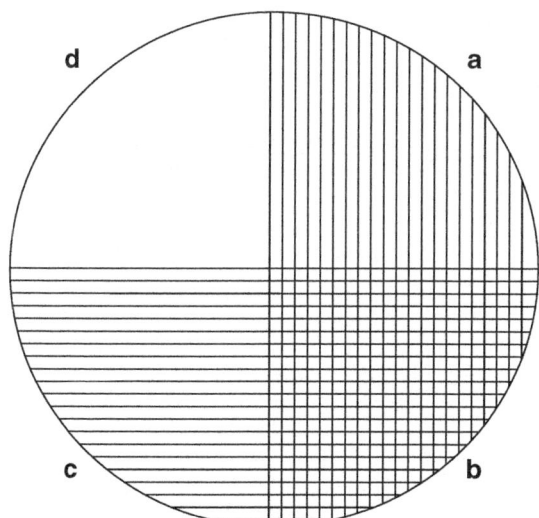

Fig. 1.1 Quadrant method for axis determination. The positive region of lead I is depicted with *vertical striping*. The positive region of aVF is shown with *horizontal striping*. By determining the orientation of lead I and aVF, the quadrant of the QRS axis can be easily determined. In quadrant *b*, both lead I and aVF are positive. In quadrant *a*, lead I is positive and aVF is negative

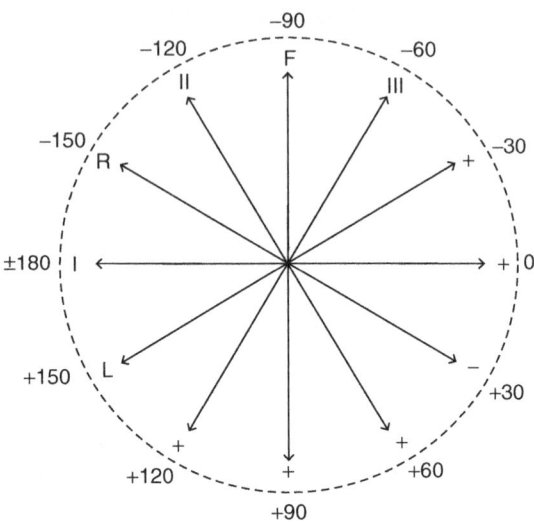

Fig. 1.2 The isolectric method of axis determination. The location of the isolectrical lead is determined from the 12-lead ECG. The axis lies perpendicular (90°) to the isolectric lead

Q–T correction:

$$\mathbf{Q} - \mathbf{T}_c = \frac{\text{measured } Q - T \text{ interval}}{\text{square root of } R - R \text{ interval}}$$

■ 9. ADVANCED CARDIAC LIFE SUPPORT ALGORITHMS (FIGS. 1.3, 1.4, 1.5, 1.6)

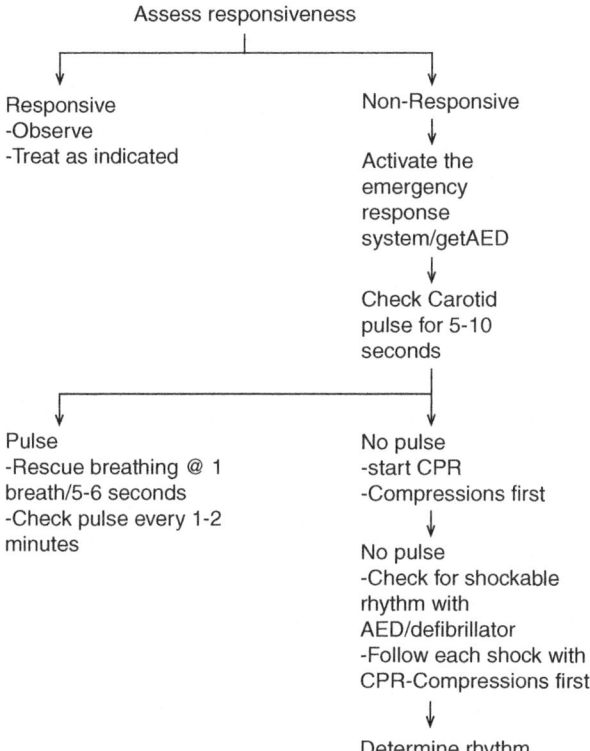

Fig. 1.3 The algorithm approach [Modified from American Heart Association. (2011). *Advanced cardiovascular life support*. American Heart Association]

a

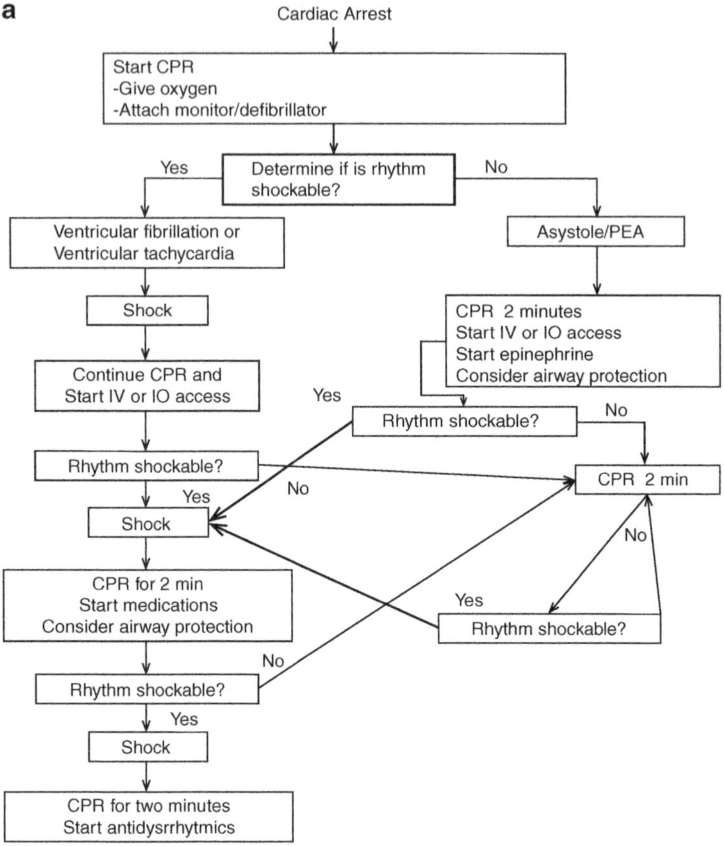

Cardiac Arrest

Start CPR
-Give oxygen
-Attach monitor/defibrillator

Yes ←── Determine if is rhythm shockable? ──→ No

Ventricular fibrillation or Ventricular tachycardia

Asystole/PEA

Shock

CPR 2 minutes
Start IV or IO access
Start epinephrine
Consider airway protection

Continue CPR and Start IV or IO access

Yes

Rhythm shockable? ──→ No

Rhythm shockable?

CPR 2 min

Yes

No

No

Shock

CPR for 2 min
Start medications
Consider airway protection

Yes

Rhythm shockable?

No

Rhythm shockable?

Yes

Shock

CPR for two minutes
Start antidysrrhytmics

b

Return of Spontaneous Circulation (ROSC)
- Pulse and blood pressure
- Abrupt sustained increased in PETCO2 (typically ≥ 40 mm Hg)

Shock Energy
- **Biphasic:** Manufacturer recommendation
- **Monophasic:** 360 J

Drug therapy
- **Epinephrine IV/IO Dose:** 1 mg q 3-5 minutes
- **Vasopressin IV/IO Dose:** 40 units
- **Amiodarone IV/IO Dose:** first dose 300 mg bolus.
  Second dose 150 mg.

Advanced Airway
- Supraglottic advanced airway or endotracheal intubation
- Confirm endotracheal tube placement with stethoscope as well as ETCO2
- Continue chest Compressions during ventilation

Fig. 1.4 (a) The algorithm for Ventricular Fibrillation/Pulseless Ventricular Tachycardia [Modified from American Heart Association. (2011). *Advanced cardiovascular life support*. American Heart Association]

Adult Immediate Post-Cardiac Arrest Care

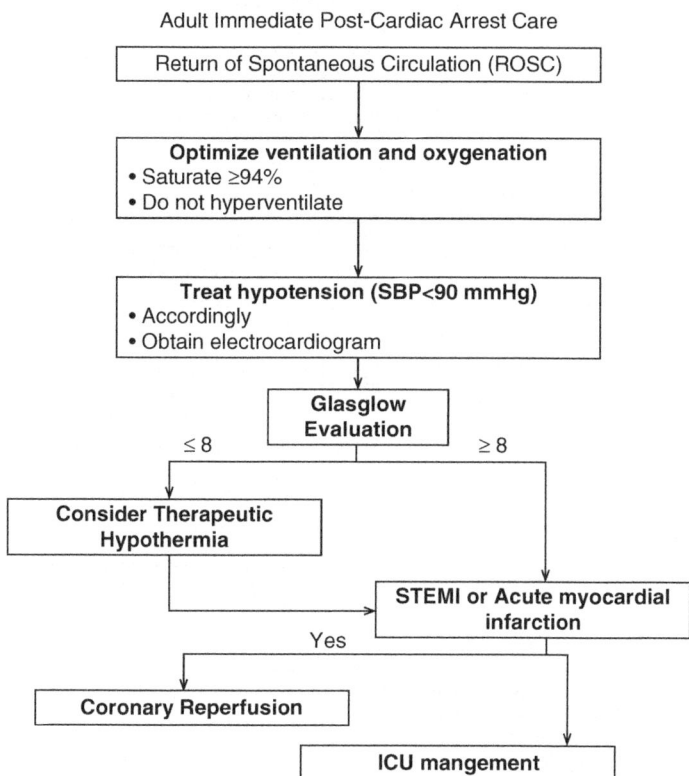

Fig. 1.5 The algorithm for Post-Cardiac Arrest Care [Modified from American Heart Association. (2011). *Advanced cardiovascular life support*. American Heart Association]

a

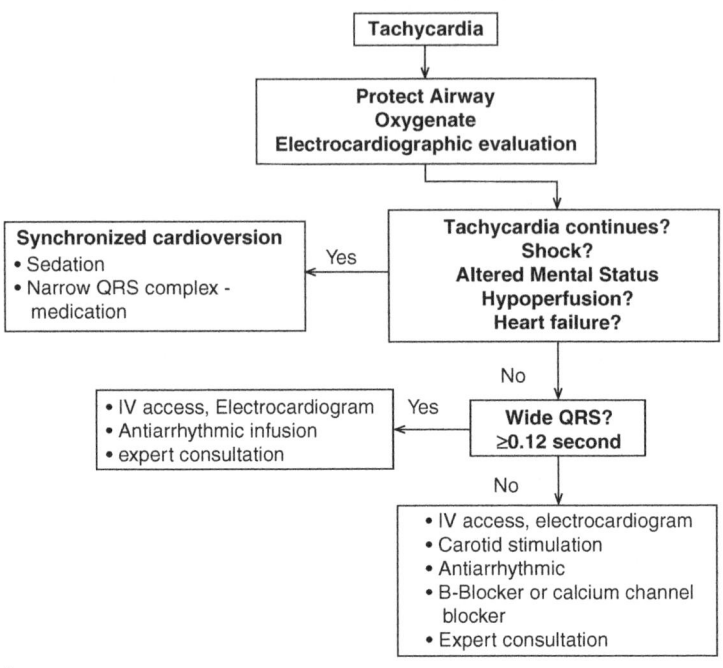

Adult tachycardia (with pulse)

Tachycardia

Protect Airway
Oxygenate
Electrocardiographic evaluation

Tachycardia continues?
Shock?
Altered Mental Status
Hypoperfusion?
Heart failure?

Yes →

Synchronized cardioversion
• Sedation
• Narrow QRS complex - medication

No ↓

Wide QRS?
≥0.12 second

Yes →

• IV access, Electrocardiogram
• Antiarrhythmic infusion
• expert consultation

No ↓

• IV access, electrocardiogram
• Carotid stimulation
• Antiarrhythmic
• B-Blocker or calcium channel blocker
• Expert consultation

b

Doses/Details

Synchronized Cardioversion
Initial recommended doses:
• Narrow regular: 50-100J
• Narrow irregular: 120-200 J biphasic or 200 J monophasic
• Wide regular: 100J
• Wide irregular: defibrillation dose (NOT synchronized)

Adenosine IV Dose:
First dose: 6 mg rapid IV push; follow with NS flush
May use double dose, if persistent

Antiarrhythmic Infusions for Stable Wide-QRS Tachycardia

Procainamide IV Dose:
20-50 mg/min until arrhythmia suppressed, hypotension ensues, QRS duration increases > 50%, or maximum dose 17 mg/kg given. Maintenance infusion: 1-4 mg/min
Avoid if prolonged QT or CHF

Amiodarone IV Dose:
First dose: 150 mg over 10 minutes. Follow by maintenance infusion of 1 mg/min for first 6 hours.

Sotalol IV Dose
100 mg (1.5 mg/kg) over 5 minutes. Avoid if prolonged QT

Fig. 1.6 (**a**) The algorithm for Adult Tachycardia with pulse. [Modified from American Heart Association. (2011). *Advanced cardiovascular life support.* American Heart Association]

■ 10. COMMON DYSRHYTHMIAS (1.7, 1.8, 1.9, 1.10, 1.11, AND 1.12)

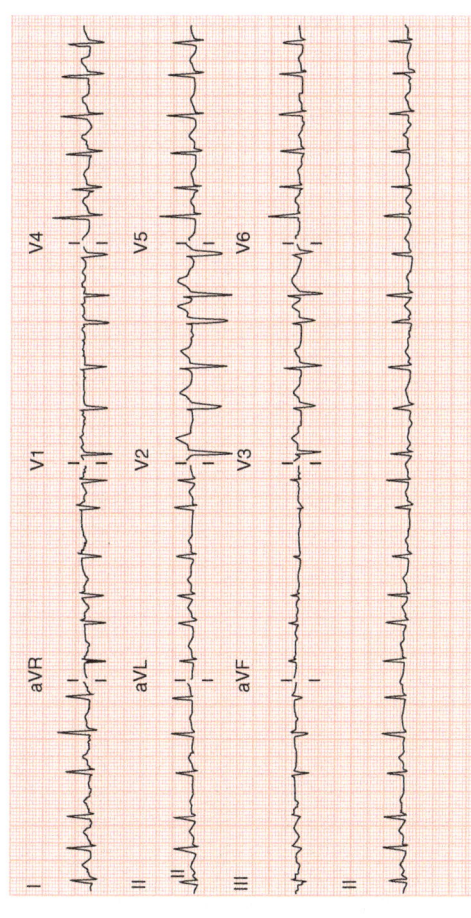

Fig 1.7 Atrial fibrillation

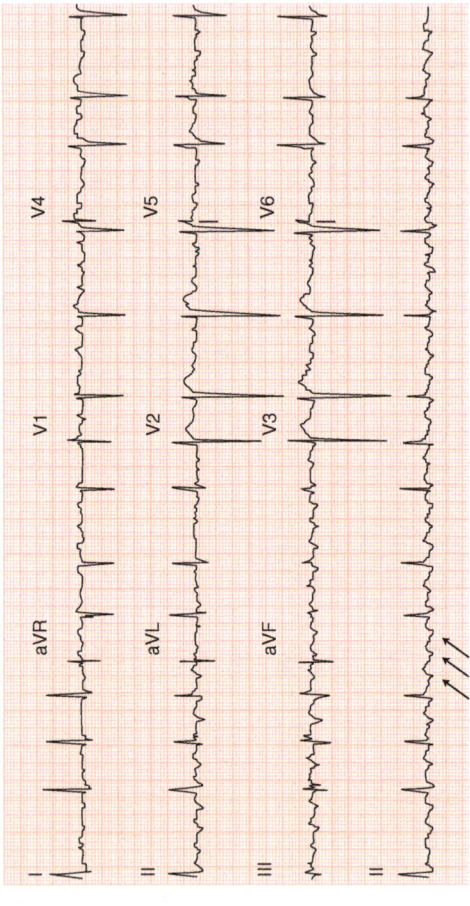

Fig. 1.8 Atrial flutter with variable block (alternating 2:1 and 3:1)

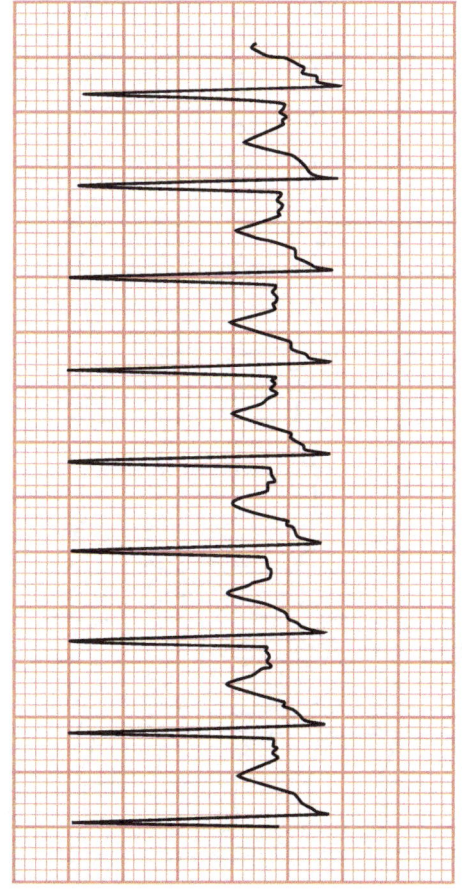

Fig. 1.9 Supraventricular tachycardia

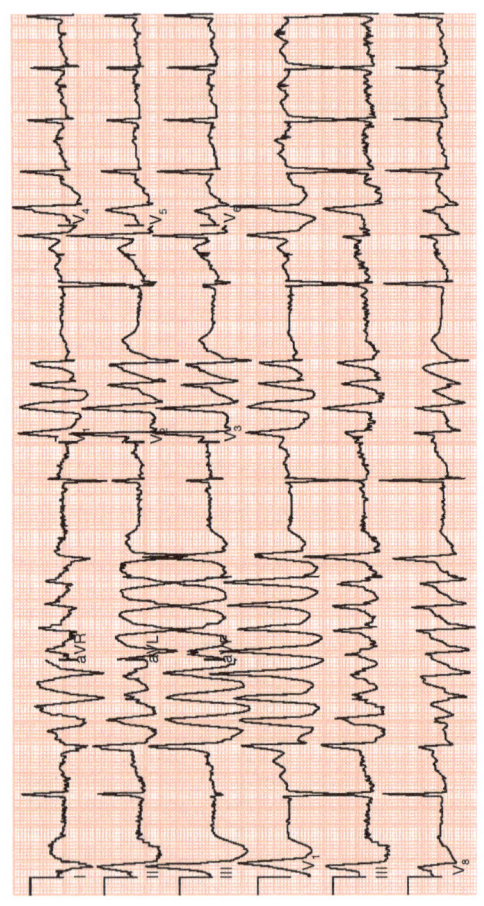

Fig. 1.10 Torsades de pointes

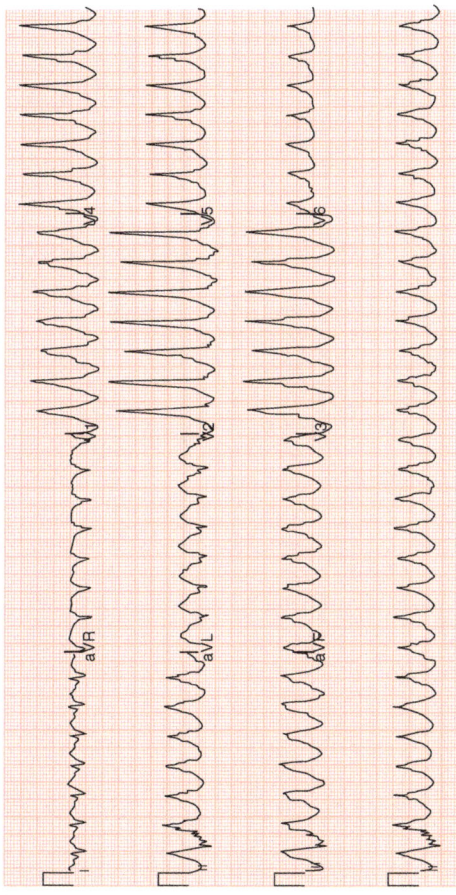

Fig. 1.11 Ventricular tachycardia

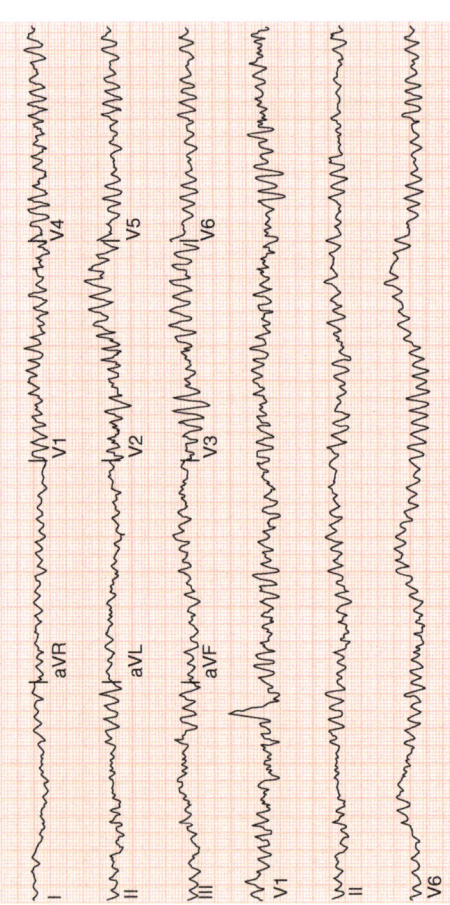

Fig. 1.12 Ventricular fibrillation

■ 11. OTHER FORMULAS AND CLASSIFICATIONS

The *New York Heart Association Functional (NYHA) Classification* (Table 1.6) is used to categorize patients by the severity of their cardiac dysfunction.

Table 1.6 New York heart association functional classification

NYHA functional classification	
I	No symptoms and no limitation in ordinary physical activity, e.g., shortness of breath when walking, climbing stairs
II	Mild symptoms (mild shortness of breath and/or angina) and slight limitation during ordinary activity
III	Marked limitation in activity due to symptoms, even during less than ordinary activity, e.g., walking short distances 20–100 m. Comfortable only at rest
IV	Severe limitation. Experiences symptoms even while at rest. Mostly bedbound patients

2

Endocrinology and Metabolism Facts and Formulas

Alterations in endocrinology and metabolism are common in critically ill patients. Laboratory testing and interpretation of laboratory data play an important part in the management of these disorders.

■ 1. ADRENAL FUNCTION

The question of adrenal insufficiency in critical ill patients arises commonly.

Normal serum cortisol levels vary during the day in normal individuals, the reference ranges are:

– Highest in the early morning 7–8 mcg/dL
– Lowest in the afternoon 2–18 mcg/dL

Blood sample taken at 8 in the morning are 6–23 (mcg/dL).

Formal *ACTH stimulation test* (may be measured while administering dexamethasone 10 mg I.V q6hrs):

– Baseline cortisol
– 0.25 mg Corticotropin I.V. or I.M.
– Cortisol level at 60 min
– <7 mcg/dL increase after doing the ACTH stimulation test suggests primary adrenal insufficiency if the basal cortisol level is <20 mcg/dL

Corticosteroids are commonly used in inflammatory disorders and for replacement therapy. Equivalent doses are shown in Table 2.1:

J. Varon and R.E. Fromm Jr., *Acute and Critical Care Formulas and Laboratory Values*, DOI 10.1007/978-1-4614-7510-1_2, © Springer Science+Business Media New York 2014

Table 2.1 Equivalent corticosteroid doses

Agent	Dose (mg)	Duration (h)	Potency	
			Mineralocorticoid	Glucocorticoid
Cortisol	20.0	8	1.0	1.0
Cortisone	25.0	8	1.0	0.8
Dexamethasone	0.75	72	0	25
Hydrocortisone	20.0	8	1.0	0.8
Methylprednisolone	4.0	36	0.5	5
Prednisolone	5.0	24	0.8	4
Prednisone	5.0	24	0.8	4

■ 2. DIABETES INSIPIDUS (DI)

A disorder of fluid homeostasis because of inadequate antidiuretic hormone (ADH) secretion or action:

Neurogenic DI = Inadequate production or secretion of ADH

Nephrogenic DI = Unresponsiveness of renal tubules to ADH

Water Deprivation Test
The *water deprivation test* (Table 2.2) may be performed if the patient is hemodynamically stable and the serum sodium is <145 mEq/L:

Table 2.2 Water deprivation test

	Maximum U_{osm} (mOsm/ kg H_2O)	Maximum U_{osm} P_{osm}	% Change after vasopressin[a]	Maximum U_{osm}/P_{osm} after vasopressin[a]
Normal	800–1,200	>1	<9 %	>1
Partial diabetes insipidus	400	>1	>9 %	>1
Complete diabetes insipidus	100–200	<1	>50 %	Variable
Nephrogenic diabetes insipidus	<150	<1	<45 %	<1

[a]5 U subcutaneously

■ 3. SODIUM FORMULAS

Serum Sodium Correction in Hyperglycemia

$$Na^+ = \text{Measured } Na^+ + 0.016 \text{ (serum glucose} - 100)$$

Serum Sodium Correction in Hyperlipidemia and Hyperproteinemia

Decrease (mEq / L) serum Na^+ in hyperlipidemia $= \text{Plasma lipids (mg / dL)} \times 0.002$

Decrease (mEq / L) serum Na^+ in hyperlipidemia $= 0.25* \text{(protein (g / dL))}$

Estimated Sodium Excess in Hypernatremia

Na^+ excess (mEq / L) $= 0.6 \text{ body weight (kg)} \times \text{(current plasma } Na^+ - 140)$

Estimated Sodium Deficit in Hyponatremia

Na^+ deficit (mEq) $= 0.6 \times \text{body weight} \times$
$$\text{(desired plasma } Na^+ - \text{current plasma } Na^+)$$

■ 4. OSMOLALITY FORMULAS

$$\textbf{Calculated osmolality} = 2(Na^+) + \frac{\text{Glucose}}{18} + \frac{\text{BUN}}{2.8}$$

$$\textbf{Effective osmolality} = 2(Na^+) + \frac{\text{Glucose}}{18}$$

Osmolal gap $= \text{Measured osmolality} - \text{calculated osmolality}$

■ 5. DIABETES MELLITUS

Complications of diabetes mellitus may be the presenting condition of a patient in the ICU. However, many other patients may develop glucose intolerance while in the ICU.

Diabetic ketoacidosis (DKA) and non-ketotic hyperosmolar coma (HNKC) may present similarly. The following characteristics (see Table 2.3) may help the clinician differentiate between the two:

Table 2.3 Laboratory presentation of DKA and HNKC

Laboratory test	DKA	HNKC
Blood glucose (mg/dL)	200–2,000	Usually > 600
Blood ketones	Present	Absent
Arterial pH	<7.4	Normal[a]
Anion gap	↑↑	Normal or ↑↑
Osmolality	↑	↑↑
Urine dipstick	Glucose and ketones	Glucose

DKA = diabetic ketoacidosis; HNKC = Hyperglycemic non-ketotic coma;
↑ = slightly elevated; ↑↑ = elevated
[a]May be low if hypovolemia causes poor tissue perfusion

Table 2.4 contains some of the insulins commonly employed in the ICU setting:

Table 2.4 Types of insulins commonly employed in the ICU

Type of insulin	Onset of action (min)	Peak (min)	Duration (min)
Regular (I.V.)	5	20–25	40–45
Regular (I.M.)	30	60	90–100
Regular (S.Q.)	60	180	360
NPH (S.Q.)	240	360–480	600–960
Lente (S.Q.)	240	360–480	600–960
Ultralente (S.Q.)	480–720	720–1,080	1,080–1,680

■ 6. HYPOGLYCEMIA (TABLE 2.5)

Table 2.5 Differentiating exogenous insulin administration, insulinoma, and oral hypoglycemic agent-induced hypoglycemia

Laboratory test	Insulinoma	Exogenous insulin	Sulfonylureas	Insulin autoimmune
Plasma insulin level	↑	↑↑	↑	↑
Insulin antibodies	None[a]	Present	None[a]	↓
Plasma/urine sulfonylurea levels	Absent	Absent	Present	Absent
C-peptide	↑	N/↓	↑	↑

Other causes of hypoglycemia such as hepatic failure should be considered in the ICU
↑ = increased; ↓ = decreased; N = normal
[a]May be present if the patient has had prior insulin injections

■ 7. THYROID FUNCTION TESTS (TABLES 2.6 AND 2.7)

Table 2.6 Thyroid function tests

Direct methods	Indirect methods
Circulating levels of total hormones:	*Thyroid hormone binding test:*
Total thyroxine (T_4)	Resin uptake of ^{125}I–T_3
Total triiodothyronine (T_3)	
Protein-bound iodine (PBI)	
Circulating levels of free hormones:	*Free thyroxine index (FTI):*
Free thyroxine (fT_4)	$$\mathbf{FTI} = \frac{T_4 \times \text{patient triiodothyronine } (T_3)}{\text{Control triiodothyronine } (T_3)}$$
Free triiodothyronine (fT_3)	
Thyroid hormone-binding proteins:	
Thyroxine-binding globulin (TBG)	

Table 2.7 Interpretation of thyroid function tests in the ICU

Test	Hypothyroid	High T_4 syndrome	Hyperthyroid	Low T_3 syndrome	Low T_3/T_4 syndrome
TSH	High[a]	Nl/low	Low	Low to sl ↑	Low to sl ↑
Total T_4	Low	High	High	Nl	Low
Total T_3	Low to low Nl	Low/Nl/high	High	Low	Low
Reverse T_3	Nl/low	Nl/high	High	High	High
Free T_4	Low	Nl/high	High	Nl	Nl
T_3RU	Low	Nl/low	High	Nl/high	High

Nl=normal; *sl*= slight
[a]Except TSH is low in hypothyroidism of secondary and tertiary causes

■ **8. CALCIUM METABOLISM AND DISORDERS**

$$\textbf{Corrected Ca}^{++} = \text{Measured Ca}^{++} + 0.8 \times (4 - \text{plasma albumin})$$

$$\textbf{Corrected Ca}^{++} \textbf{ (quick method)} = \text{Ca}^{++} - \text{albumin} + 4$$

In the differential diagnosis of hypercalcemia, the use of urinary cyclic AMP and parathyroid hormone may confirm a diagnosis (see Table 2.8):

Table 2.8 Use of iPTH and urinary cyclic AMP in the differential diagnosis of hypercalcemia

iPTH	Urinary cyclic AMP	iPLP	Diagnosis
↑ ↑	↑ ↑	N	Primary hyperparathyroidism
N or ↓	N or ↓	↑	Probable occult malignancy

↑ =increased; ↓ =decreased; *N*=normal
iPTH= Parathyroid hormone by radioimmunoassay; *iPLP*=parathyroid hormone-like protein by radioimmunoassay

■ 9. NUTRITION FORMULAS

Please refer to Chap. 8 for additional formulas.

Body Mass Index
The *body mass index* (BMI) is frequently utilized when dealing with nutrition in the critically ill patient:

$$\mathbf{BMI} = \frac{(\text{Body weight [kg]})}{(\text{Height [m]}^2)}$$

Harris–Benedict Equation
It measures the basal energy expenditure (BEE), which represents the resting basal metabolic rate:

Men:

$$66 + (13.7 \times W) + (\% \times H) - (5.0 \times A) = \text{kcal / day}$$

Women:

$$655 + (9.6 \times W) + (1.85 \times H) - (4.7 \times A) = \text{kcal / day}$$

where

W = body weight in kilograms

H = height in centimeters

A = age in years

Nitrogen Balance (NB)
Requires knowledge of protein intake urine urea nitrogen (UUN). For patients with normal renal function, the following formula is utilized:

$$\mathbf{NB} = (\text{Dietary protein} \times 0.16) - (\text{UUN} + 2 \text{ g stool} + 2 \text{ g skin})$$

In patients with renal dysfunction, the increased blood urea pool and extrarenal losses must be accounted for, and the following formula is used:

$$\mathbf{NB} = \text{Nitrogen in} - (\text{UUN} + 2 \text{ g stool} + 2 \text{ g skin} + \text{BUN change})$$

Catabolic Index (CI)
The *catabolic index* (CI) is derived from the same variables:

$$\mathbf{CI} = \text{UUN} - [(0.5 \times \text{dietary protein} \times 0.16) + 3 \text{ g}]$$

3

Environmental Facts and Formulas

Physical factors such as temperature, pressure, altitude, and humidity affect gases in particular and, thus, should be well understood by the critical care practitioner. A number of useful tables, formulas, and figures follow. Thermal injuries are commonly considered environmental events, and, thus, these formulas and figures are included in this chapter as well.

■ 1. TEMPERATURE

Temperature conversion calculations are often done in the management of critically ill patients. Degrees *Celsius* (°C) and *Fahrenheit* (°F) are most commonly utilized:

°C to °F

$$°\mathbf{F} = (°C \times 9/5) + 32$$

°F to °C

$$°\mathbf{C} = (°F - 32) \times 5/9$$

Occasionally, the *Kelvin* (K) temperature scale is used, primarily in gas law calculations:

K to °C

$$\mathbf{K} = °C + 273$$

°C to K

$$°\mathbf{C} = K - 273$$

J. Varon and R.E. Fromm Jr., *Acute and Critical Care Formulas and Laboratory Values*, DOI 10.1007/978-1-4614-7510-1_3, © Springer Science+Business Media New York 2014

■ 2. HUMIDITY

Relative Humidity
Relative humidity (RH) is usually measured by hygrometers, thus eliminating the
need of extracting and measuring the humidity content of the air samples:

$$\mathbf{RH} = \frac{\text{Content [mg / L or mm Hg]}}{\text{Capacity [mg / L or mm Hg]}} = \%$$

Humidity Deficit
The *humidity deficit* (HD) represents the maximum humidity capacity at body
temperature:

$$\mathbf{HD} = \text{Capacity} - \text{content} = \text{mg / L}$$

where

   capacity=amount of water the alveolar air can hold at body temperature (also
      known as absolute humidity)
   content=humidity content of inspired air (see Table 3.1):

Table 3.1 Humidity capacity of saturated gases from 0 to 43 °C

Gas temperature (°C)	Water content (mg/L)	Water vapor pressure (mmHg)
0	4.9	4.6
5	6.8	6.6
10	9.4	9.3
17	14.5	14.6
18	15.4	15.6
19	16.3	16.5
20	17.3	17.5
21	18.4	18.7
22	19.4	19.8
23	20.6	21.1
24	21.8	22.4
25	23.1	23.8

(continued)

Table 3.1 (continued)

Gas temperature (°C)	Water content (mg/L)	Water vapor pressure (mmHg)
26	24.4	25.2
27	25.8	26.7
28	27.2	28.3
29	28.8	30.0
30	30.4	31.8
31	32.0	33.7
32	33.8	35.7
33	35.6	37.7
34	37.6	39.9
35	39.6	42.2
36	41.7	44.6
37	43.9	47.0
38	46.2	49.8
39	48.6	52.5
40	51.1	55.4
41	53.7	58.4
42	56.5	61.6

■ **3. PRESSURE**

Pressure is defined as force per unit area, and there are various ways of measuring this force. One way is that force can be recorded in a form of the height of a column as in the mercury barometer; therefore, it can be recorded in milliliters of mercury (mmHg) pressure or centimeters of water pressure.

To Convert cmH_2O *to* mmHg

$$\mathbf{mmHg} = cmH_2O \times 0.735$$

To Convert mmHg *to* cmH_2O

$$\mathbf{cmH_2O} = mmHg \times 1.36$$

Pressure Per Square Inch

A less commonly used conversion in clinical medicine includes converting *Psi (pressure per square inch) to mmHg*:

$$\mathbf{mmHg} = \text{Psi} \times 51.7$$

Pressure-Related Formulas

Other useful pressure-related formulas/facts include:

$$\textbf{Total pressure} = P_1 + P_2 + P_3 + \cdots \text{(Dalton's Law)}$$

$$\textbf{1 atmosphere} = 760 \text{ mmHg} = 29.921 \text{ in Hg} = 33.93 \text{ ft H}_2\text{O} = 1{,}034 \text{ cm H}_2\text{O}$$
$$= 1{,}034 \text{ g / cm}^2 = 14.7 \text{ lb / in.}^2$$

Pressure/Volume Relationships

Useful pressure/volume relationships that can be used in the management of critically ill patients include:

$$\textbf{Volume}_{\text{BTPS}} = \text{Volume}_{\text{ATPS}} \times \text{Factor}$$

where

Volume$_{\text{BTPS}}$ = gas volume saturated with water at body temperature (37 °C) and ambient pressure [BTPS = barometric temperature pressure saturation]

Volume$_{\text{ATPS}}$ = gas volume saturated with water at ambient (room) temperature and pressure [ATPS = ambient temperature pressure saturation]

Factor represents the factors for converting gas volumes from ATPS to BTPS:

$$\textbf{Conversion factor} = \frac{P_\text{B} - P\text{H}_2\text{O}}{P_\text{B} - 47} \times \frac{310}{\left(273 + °\text{ C}\right)}$$

See also Table 3.2:

Table 3.2 Factors for converting gas volumes from ATPS to BTPS

Gas temperature (°C)	Factors to convert to 37 °C saturated	Water vapor pressure (mmHg)
18	1.112	15.6
19	1.107	16.5
20	1.102	17.5
21	1.096	18.7
22	1.091	19.8
23	1.085	21.1
24	1.080	22.4
25	1.075	23.8
26	1.068	25.2
27	1.063	26.7
28	1.057	28.3
29	1.051	30.0
30	1.045	31.8
31	1.039	33.7
32	1.032	35.7
33	1.026	37.7
34	1.020	39.9
35	1.014	42.2
36	1.007	44.6
37	1.000	47.0
38	0.993	49.8
39	0.986	52.5
40	0.979	55.4
41	0.971	58.4
42	0.964	61.6

■ 4. ALTITUDE

As altitude varies, changes in atmospheric pressure produce alterations in gas density (see Table 3.3):

Table 3.3 Changes in density with altitude assuming a constant temperature

Altitude (ft)	Standard temperature (°C)	Density ratio constant temperature	Density ratio standard temperature
0	15.00	1.0000	1.0000
5,000	5.09	0.8320	0.8617
10,000	−4.81	0.6877	0.7385
15,000	−14.72	0.5643	0.6292

■ 5. BURNS

To estimate the extent of burn, the *rule of nines* for body surface area (BSA) is commonly used:

Adults: Arms 9 % each; legs 18 % each; head 9 %; trunk 18 % anterior, 18 % posterior; genitalia 1 %.

Children: Arms 9 % each; legs 16 % each; head 13 %; trunk 18 % anterior, 18 % posterior; genitalia 1 %.

Infants: Arms 9 % each; legs 14 % each; head 18 %; trunk 18 % anterior, 18 % posterior; genitalia 1 %.

In addition, the *Lund and Browder chart* (Fig. 3.1) can be used (more accurate in children).

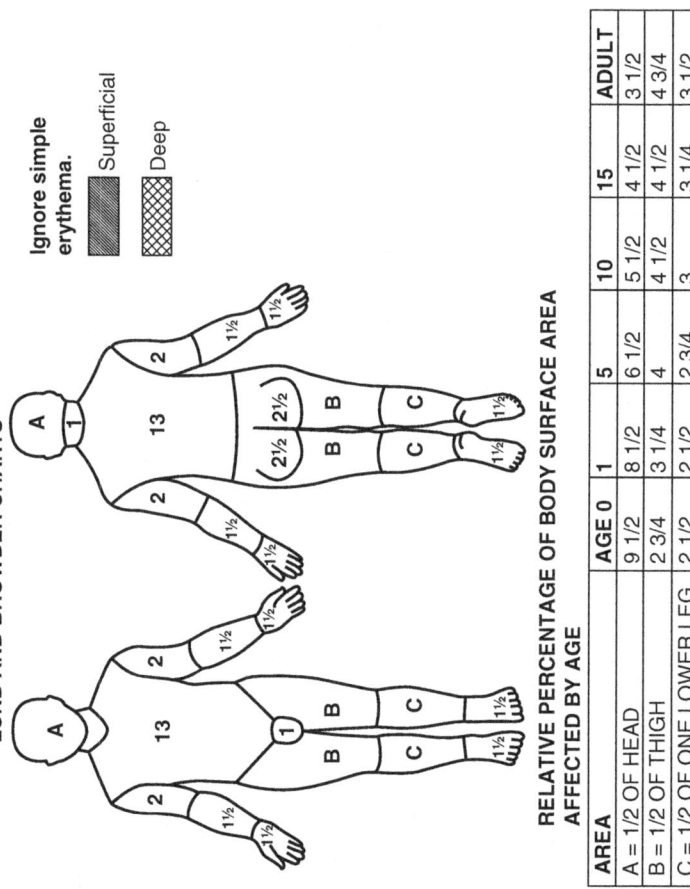

LUND AND BROWDER CHARTS

Ignore simple erythema.

▨ Superficial

▩ Deep

RELATIVE PERCENTAGE OF BODY SURFACE AREA AFFECTED BY AGE

AREA	AGE 0	1	5	10	15	ADULT
A = 1/2 OF HEAD	9 1/2	8 1/2	6 1/2	5 1/2	4 1/2	3 1/2
B = 1/2 OF THIGH	2 3/4	3 1/4	4	4 1/2	4 1/2	4 3/4
C = 1/2 OF ONE LOWER LEG	2 1/2	2 1/2	2 3/4	3	3 1/4	3 1/2

Fig. 3.1 Lund and Browder chart for estimation of burn extent

4

Gastrointestinal Facts and Formulas

Problems of the gastrointestinal system commonly result in ED visits and ICU admissions. In addition, critically ill patients may suffer from stress-induced mucosal injury, ileus, and hepatic dysfunction. The following formulas and facts should be useful in a broad range of ICU patients and patients presenting to the ED. Many additional important facts and formulas related to the GI tract can be found in Chap. 8.

■ 1. INTESTINAL TRANSIT

The normal 24-h *intestinal fluid and electrolyte transport* is depicted in Table 4.1:

■ 2. STOOL FORMULAS

As part of the diagnostic work-up of patients with diarrhea, *stool osmolal gap* (SOG) is usually calculated utilizing the following formula:

$$\mathbf{SOG} = \text{stool osmolality} - 2 \times (\text{stool Na}^+ + \text{stool K}^+)$$

Normal stool osmolality is <290 mOsm/L. If the SOG > 100, it indicates an osmotic diarrhea and <100 indicates secretory diarrhea.

J. Varon and R.E. Fromm Jr., *Acute and Critical Care Formulas and Laboratory Values*, DOI 10.1007/978-1-4614-7510-1_4, © Springer Science+Business Media New York 2014

Table 4.1 Normal 24-h intestinal fluid and electrolyte transport

Site	Fluid received (L)	Amount absorbed (L)	Electrolyte absorption		
			Na^+	K^+	Cl^-
Duodenum/ jejunum	9.0	4.0	Passive	Passive	Passive
Ileum	5.0	3.5	Active	Passive	Passive
Colon	1.5	1.35	Active	Passive	Active

■ **3. LIVER FACTS**

Child–Pugh Classification
The *Child–Pugh classification* for portal hypertension is commonly used in critically ill patients and is depicted in Table 4.2:

Table 4.2 Child–Pugh classification of portal hypertension

Class	A	B	C
Serum bilirubin (mg/dL)	<2	2–3	>3
Serum albumin (g/dL)	>3.5	3–3.5	<3
Ascites	None	Easily controlled	Poorly controlled
Encephalopathy	None	Minimal	Advanced
Nutrition	Excellent	Good	Poor

■ **4. HEPATITIS**

The interpretation of laboratory tests performed in patients with *viral hepatitis* is depicted in Table 4.3.

Table 4.3 Common hepatitis screening laboratory tests

Test	Positive results indicates
• ALT elevation	• Hepatocyte injury and can occur in acute or chronic hepatitis and other types of liver disease. Patients with severe cirrhosis may have ALT levels which fall within the normal range
• Anti-HAV–IgM • Anti-HAV–Total or Anti-HAV–IgG	• Acute hepatitis A infection • Immunity to hepatitis A from natural infection if anti-HAV–IgM is nonreactive. Can be false negative after vaccination
• HBsAg • Anti-HBc–IgM • Anti-HBc–total (IgM+IgG) • Anti-HBs • HBeAg, anti-HBe, HBV DNA	• Hepatitis B virus infection and infectiousness • Acute or chronic hepatitis B infection (about 20 % of chronic HBV infected people display anti-HBc–IgM) • Infection with hepatitis B does not imply immunity • Immunity to hepatitis B, due to vaccination. If both anti-HBcTotal and anti-HBs reactive (and HBsAg is nonreactive) this indicates resolved hepatitis B infection • Useful for hepatitis B monitoring
• Anti-HCV • HCV RNA	• Indicates exposure to hepatitis C. Does not imply immunity, usually represents active infection (confirm by testing for HCV RNA) • Presence of hepatitis C virus infection

5

Hematological Facts and Formulas

Patients in the emergency department and the intensive care unit frequently have hematologic problems. These include anemia, coagulopathies, and thrombocytopenia to name just a few. In evaluation these patients, many laboratory tests and indices are obtained. The following formulas will aid the critical care practitioner in evaluating these hematologic parameters.

■ 1. RED BLOOD CELLS

Mean Corpuscular Volume
The *mean corpuscular volume* (MCV) indicates the average volume of a single RBC in a given blood sample and is calculated as:

$$\text{MCV} = \frac{\text{Hct } (\%) \times 10}{\text{RBC } (10^{12} / \text{L})}$$

Mean Corpuscular Hemoglobin
The *mean corpuscular hemoglobin* (MCH) indicates the average weight of Hb per erythrocyte:

$$\text{MCH} = \frac{\text{Hb } (\text{g} / \text{dL}) \times 10}{\text{RBC } (10^{12} / \text{L})}$$

J. Varon and R.E. Fromm Jr., *Acute and Critical Care Formulas and Laboratory Values*, DOI 10.1007/978-1-4614-7510-1_5, © Springer Science+Business Media New York 2014

Mean Corpuscular Hemoglobin Concentration
The *mean corpuscular hemoglobin concentration* (MCHC) indicates the average concentration of Hb in the RBCs of any specimen:

$$\mathbf{MCHC} = \frac{\text{Hb (g / dL)}}{\text{Hct (\%)}} \times 100$$

Red Blood Cell Volume
The *red blood cell volume* can be calculated via a radionuclide study:

$$\mathbf{RBC\ volume} = \frac{\text{cpm of isotope injected}}{\text{cpm / mL RBC in sample}}$$

where

cpm = counts per million

■ **2. RETICULOCYTES COUNT**

Percentage of Reticulocytes
To calculate the *percentage of reticulocytes* usually based on counting 1,000 RBCs, the following formula is commonly utilized:

$$\mathbf{Reticulocytes\ (\%)} = \frac{\text{Number of reticulocytes}}{\text{Number of RBC observed}} \times 100$$

Actual Reticulocyte Count
The *actual reticulocyte count* (ARC) reflects the actual number of reticulocytes in 1 L of whole blood:

$$\mathbf{ARC} = \frac{\text{Reticulocytes (\%)}}{100} \times \text{RBC count } (\times 10^{12} / \text{L}) \times 1,000$$

Corrected Reticulocyte Count
The corrected reticulocyte count (CRC) is calculated as:

$$\mathbf{CRC} = \text{Reticulocytes (\%)} \times \frac{\text{Hct (L / L)}}{0.45\,\text{L / L}}$$

Reticulocyte Production Index
The reticulocyte count is usually viewed in relation to the degree of anemia. The *reticulocyte production index* (RPI) is a frequently used correction method:

$$\mathbf{RPI} = \frac{(\text{Measured Hct / Normal Hct}) \times \text{Reticulocyte count}}{\text{Maturation time in peripheral blood}}$$

Maturation Factor
The *maturation factor* varies according to the hematocrit as shown in Table 5.1:

Table 5.1 Maturation of reticulocytes in peripheral blood

Hematocrit	Maturation time in days
0.41–0.50	1
0.30–0.40	1.5
0.20–0.39	2
0.10–0.19	2.5

A normal RPI is 1.0, an RPI of 3.0 or more represents adequate response of the marrow to anemia. An RPI of <2.0 represents an inadequate response in the presence of anemia.

■ 3. ANEMIAS

The red blood cell indices (MCV, MCHC, and MCH) (see Table 5.2) are frequently utilized to classify anemias:

Table 5.2 Red blood cell indices in hypochromic and microcytic anemias

	MCV (fl)	MCHC (g/dL)	MCH (pg)
Normal	83–96	32–36	28–34
Hypochromic	83–100	28–31	23–31
Microcytic	70–82	32–36	22–27
Hypochromic–microcytic	50–79	24–31	11–29

Table 5.3 depicts the laboratory *differentiation of microcytic anemias*:

Table 5.3 Differentiation of microcytic anemias

Abnormality	Ferritin	Serum iron	TIBC	RDW
Chronic disease	N/↑	↓	↓	N
Iron deficiency	↓	↓	↑	↑
Sideroblastic anemia	N/↑	↑	N	N
Thalassemia	N/↑	N/↑	N	N/↑

N=Normal; ↑=increased; ↓=decreased; *TIBC*=total iron binding capacity; *RDW*=red cell distribution width

■ 4. HEMOLYTIC DISORDERS

Table 5.4 depicts some of the common RBC morphological abnormalities encountered in patients with *hemolytic disorders*:

Table 5.4 Red blood cells morphological abnormalities in hemolytic disorders

Abnormality	Hemolytic disorder	
	Congenital	Acquired
Fragmented cells (schistocytes)	Unstable hemoglobins (Heinz body anemias)	Microangiopathic processes
		Prosthetic heart valves
		Disseminated intravascular coagulation
		Thrombotic thrombocytopenic purpura
Permanently sickled cells	Sickle cell anemia	
Spur cells (acanthocytes)	Abetalipoproteinemia	Severe liver disease
Spherocytes	Hereditary spherocytosis	Immune, warm-antibody type
Target cells	Thalassemia	Liver disease
	Hemoglobinopathies (Hb C)	Splenectomy
Agglutinated cells		Immune, cold agglutinin disease

■ 5. HUMAN HEMOGLOBINS

Table 5.5 depicts the normal human hemoglobins at different stages of life:

Table 5.5 Normal human hemoglobins at different stages of life

Hemoglobin	Molecular structure	Stage	Proportion (%) Newborns	Adults
Portland	$\zeta_2 \gamma_2$	Embryonic	0	0
Gower I	$\zeta_2 \varepsilon_2$	Embryonic	0	0
Gower II	$\alpha_2 \varepsilon_2$	Embryonic	0	0
Fetal (F)	$\alpha_2 \gamma_2$	Newborn/adult	80	<1
A_1	$\alpha_2 \beta_2$	Newborn/adult	20	97
A_2	$\alpha_2 \delta_2$	Newborn/adult	<0.5	2.5

To convert colorimetric readings into grams of Hb per dL (g/dL) using a standard curve setup with same equipment and reagents used for specimen or calculate specimen concentration (C_u) based on *Beer's law*, the following formula is utilized:

$$C_u \text{ (g / dL)} = 301 \frac{(A_u \times C_s)}{A_s} \times \frac{1}{1,000} = \frac{0.301 (A_u \times C_s)}{A_s}$$

where

A_u = absorbance of the unknown
C_s = concentration of the standard (usually 80 mg/dL)
A_s = absorbance of the standard run most recently under the same conditions as the patient specimen

Hemoglobin F
To calculate the fraction of *hemoglobin F as a percentage*, the following formula is used:

$$\textbf{Hb F (\%)} = \frac{A_{\text{test}}}{A_{\text{diluted total}} \times 5} \times 100$$

where

A = absorbance
5 = additional dilution factor

Hemoglobin A$_2$
To calculate the *percentage of hemoglobin A$_2$*:

$$\text{Hb A}_2 \text{ (\% of total)} = \frac{A \text{ fraction I}}{A \text{ fraction I} + (2.5 \times [A \text{ fraction II}])} \times 100\%$$

where

A fraction I = absorbance at 415 nm of Hb A$_2$ eluate after diluting to 10 mL volume

A fraction II = absorbance at 415 nm of eluate (after diluting to 25 mL volume) containing all other hemoglobins after Hb A$_2$ has been eluted (multiplying by a factor of 2.5 corrects for the difference in dilution volumes between fractions I and II).

■ 6. EOSINOPHILS

Absolute Direct Eosinophil Count
To calculate the *absolute direct eosinophil count*, the following formula can be employed:

$$\text{Eosinophils } (\times 10^9 / \text{L}) = \frac{\text{Eosinophil count} \times \text{Dilution factor}}{\text{Volume counted (mm}^3) \times 10^6}$$

■ 7. ACQUIRED INHIBITORS

Occasional in the ICU patients present acquired inhibitors. The titer of the inhibitors is represented by Bethesda units (BU):

$$\textbf{1 BU} = \text{inhibits 1 unit of factor VIII}$$

To calculate the amount of factor VIII required to neutralize the inhibitor and achieve a 50 % normal level of circulating factor VIII in a patient who weights 70 kg and has a plasma volume of 2,800 mL and an inhibitor titer of 10 BU/mL, the amount is:

$$\textbf{2,800 mL} \times \textbf{10.5 BU / mL} = 29,400 \text{ BU}$$

Another recommended therapy is to start with an intravenous bolus of 20 IU/kg for each BU of the inhibitor +40 addition IU/kg and monitoring FVIII levels 10 min after.

■ 8. OTHER FORMULAS

Transferrin Saturation
To calculate the *transferrin saturation*, the following formula can be applied:

$$\% \textbf{ Transferrin Saturation} = \frac{\text{Serum Iron}}{\text{TIBC}} \times 100$$

Microscopic Cell Counting
For *microscopic cell counting*, a Neubauer hemocytometer is needed and the calculation is performed as follows:

$$\textbf{Cells } (\times 10^9 / \textbf{L}) = \frac{\text{Total cells counted} \times \text{Specimen dilution factor}}{\text{mm}^2 \text{ counted} \times 0.1 \text{ mm}} \times 10^6$$

Plasma Volume
The *plasma volume* is calculated according to the equation:

$$\textbf{Plasma volume} = \frac{\text{cpm of labeled albumin injected}}{\text{cpm mL plasma at 0 h}}$$

HEMORR₂HAGES Score
The *HEMORR₂HAGES Score* (*H*epatic or renal disease, *E*thanol abuse, *M*alignancy, *O*lder, *R*educed platelet count or function, *R*e-bleeding, *H*ypertension, *A*nemia, *G*enetic factors, *E*xcessive fall risk, *S*troke) is used to predict hemorrhage in patients with atrial fibrillation as depicted in Table 5.6:

Table 5.6 The HEMORR₂HAGES score

Characteristic	Points
Prior mayor bleed	2
Hepatic or renal disease	1
Alcohol abuse	1
Malignancy	1
Age ≥75 years	1
Uncontrolled hypertension	1
Anemia	1
Excessive fall risk	1
Prior stroke	1
Reduced platelet count or fracture	1

The points are summed and then classified into the bleeding risk shown in Table 5.7.

Table 5.7 The HEMORR$_2$HAGES Score expected bleeding risk (percentage)

Points	Bleeding risk (%)
0	1.9
1	2.5
2	5.3
3	8.4
4	10.4
≥5	12.3

6

Infectious Diseases Facts and Formulas

Sepsis and its complications is one of the leading diagnosis encountered in the critical care setting. The following formulas, facts, and laboratory values are presented as a complement to the practitioner's decisions on diagnosis and management of infectious diseases in this setting.

■ 1. ANTIBIOTIC KINETICS

The pharmacokinetics of antibiotics depends on several factors.

Volume of Distribution
The *volume of distribution* (V_D) of an antimicrobial is calculated as:

$$\mathbf{V_D} = \frac{A}{C_p}$$

where

- A = total amount of antibiotic in the body
- C_p = antibiotic plasma concentration

Minimal Plasma Concentrations
Repetitive dosing of antibiotics depends on the principle of *minimal plasma concentrations* (C_{min}):

$$\mathbf{C_{min}} = \frac{D}{(V_D)(2^n - 1)}$$

J. Varon and R.E. Fromm Jr., *Acute and Critical Care Formulas and Laboratory Values*, DOI 10.1007/978-1-4614-7510-1_6, © Springer Science+Business Media New York 2014

where

D = dose
n = dosing interval expressed in half-lives

Plasma Concentration at Steady State
The *plasma concentration at steady state* (C_{ss}) of an antimicrobial can be estimated utilizing the following formula:

$$\mathbf{C}_{ss} = \frac{\text{Dose per half-life}}{(0.693)(V_D)}$$

■ 2. ANTIBIOTIC ADJUSTMENTS

Aminoglycoside Clearance
Renal dysfunction in critically ill patients is common. In those patients receiving aminoglycosides, dosage modification is required according to the *aminoglycoside clearance:*

$$\textbf{Aminoglycoside clearance} = (C_{cr})(0.6) + 10$$

where

C_{cr} = creatinine clearance in mL/min

In order to estimate the *creatinine clearance*, the *Cockcrof and Gault formula* is utilized:

Males

$$\mathbf{C}_{cr} = \frac{(140 - \text{age}) \times \text{weight}}{S_{cr} \times 72}$$

where

S_{cr} = serum creatinine in mg/dL. In women, a correction factor of 0.85 is used to adjust this formula.

Spyker and Guerrant Method
Another modification to this formula is the *Spyker and Guerrant method*:

$$\mathbf{C}_{cr}\,(\text{mL}\,/\,\text{min}) = \frac{(140 - \text{age}) \times (1.03 - 0.053 \times \text{Cr})}{\text{Cr}}$$

■ 3. ANTIBIOTIC LEVELS

Some of the clinically employed *antibiotic levels* are depicted in Table 6.1:

Table 6.1 Selected antibiotics levels

Antibiotic	Level (µg/mL)
Amikacin	Peak 20–25 through 5–10
Gentamicin	Peak 4–8 through 1–2
Chloramphenicol	Peak 15–25 through 8–10
Tobramycin	Peak 4–8 through 1–2
Vancomycin	Peak 20–40 through 5–10

■ 4. OTHER FACTS

Some of the commonly encountered in the critical care setting *atypical mycobacteria* are depicted in Table 6.2.

Table 6.2 Selected atypical mycobacteria

Category	Runyon group	Mycobacterial species
Photochromogens	I	*M. kansasii*
		M. marinum
		M. simiae
Scotochromogens	II	*M. scrofulaceum*
		M. gordonae
		M. szulgai
Nonchromogens	III	*M. avium-intracellulare*
Rapid growers	IV	*M. fortuitum*
		M. chelonae ssp. *chelonae*
		M. chelonae ssp. *abscessus*
		M. ulcerans

7

Neurological Facts and Formulas

Neurologic illness in the emergency department and the intensive care unit may be devastating. The following formulas, facts, and laboratory values may help in the diagnosis and monitoring of neurological patients.

■ 1. CEREBROSPINAL FLUID

Normal pressures and volumes for *human* Cerebrospinal Fluid (CSF) are shown in Table 7.1:

J. Varon and R.E. Fromm Jr., *Acute and Critical Care Formulas and Laboratory Values*, DOI 10.1007/978-1-4614-7510-1_7, © Springer Science+Business Media New York 2014

Table 7.1 Normal cerebrospinal fluid pressures and volumes

CSF pressure	
Children	4.4–7.3 mmHg
Adults	8–15 mmHg (lying on side)
	16–24 mmHg (standing)
Volume	
Infants	40–60 mL
Young children	60–100 mL
Older children	80–120 mL
Adult	100–160 mL

The normal *composition of the CSF* is depicted in Table 7.2:

Table 7.2 Normal composition of the human cerebrospinal fluid

	CSF concentration (mean)
Specific gravity	1.007
Osmolality (mmol/L)	280–300
pH	7.28–7.32
PCO_2 (mmHg)	44–50
Na^+ (mmol/L)	135–150
K^+ (mmol/L)	2.6–3
Ca^{++} (mmol/L)	1–1.4
Mg^{++} (mEq/L)	2.4
Cl^- (mmol/L)	115–125
Glucose (mg/dL)	50–80
Protein (mg/dL)	15–60
Lactate dehydrogenase (U/mL)	<2–7.2

Additional normal values for CSF in humans are depicted in Table 7.3:

Table 7.3 Normal cerebrospinal fluid values

CSF parameter	Newborns	Infants, older children, and adults
Leukocyte count	<32/µL	0–3/µL/mm³
Differential white cell count	<60 % polymorphs	<1 polymorph
Proteins	48–168 mg/dL	15–45 mg/dL
Glucose	30–100 mg/dL	50–80 mg/dL
CSF: blood/glucose ratio	>0.44	>0.5

In cases of hemorrhage, the white blood cell (WBC) count of the CSF may be dramatically altered. An approximation of the *WBC in blood-contaminated CSF* may be obtained by the formula:

$$\textbf{Corrected WBC count (CSF)} = \text{WBC (CSF)} - \frac{\text{WBCs (blood)} \times \text{RBC (CSF)}}{\text{RBC (blood)}}$$

When there are many RBCs or WBCs in the CSF, the total protein of the CSF may be "*corrected*" utilizing the following formula:

$$\textbf{Protein actual} = \frac{\text{Protein}_{CSF} - \text{Protein}_{serum} \times (1 - \text{Hct}) \times \text{RBC}_{CSF}}{\text{RBC}_{blood}}$$

The suggested *initial CSF studies* in patients with coma of unknown etiology are depicted in Table 7.4:

Table 7.4 CSF studies in patients with coma of unknown etiology

Tube I:
  Cell count with differential

Tube II:
  Glucose and protein

Tube III:
  Gram's stain, acid-fast bacilli stain, routine cultures, India ink and/or cryptococcal antigen, pneumococcal antigen, Venereal Disease Research Laboratories test for syphilis, and meningitis panel

Tube IV:
  Special studies (e.g., lactic acid, rheumatoid factor, and oligo bands)

The *CSF findings according to etiologic agent* are depicted in Table 7.5:

Table 7.5 CSF findings according to etiology

Parameter	Bacterial	Tuberculosis	Viral	Fungal	Parasitic	Lyme disease
Glucose (mg/dL)	<40	<45	50–80	<50	<50	<50
Protein (mg/dL)	>50	20–1,000	~45	>45	>45	>45
WBC (cm^3)	10–300	0–4,000	10–300	10–200	>10	>10
Gram's stain	+	AFB (+)	–	–	–	Antibodies

Common CSF abnormalities in patients with *multiple sclerosis* are depicted in Table 7.6:

Table 7.6 Cerebrospinal fluid abnormalities in multiple sclerosis

	Alb	IgG/TP	IgG/Alb	IgG index	Oligoclonal banding of Ig
Multiple sclerosis	25 %	67 %	60–73 %	70–90 %	85–95 %
Normal subjects	3 %	–	3–6 %	3 %	0–7 %

Alb=albumin; IgG/TP=IgG value/total protein; Ig=immunoglobulin

The abnormalities in IgG production in these patients can be estimated by the *IgG index*:

$$\textbf{IgG index} = \frac{\text{CSF IgG / CSF albumin}}{\text{Serum IgG / serum albumin}} = \text{normal} < 0.66$$

■ 2. CEREBRAL BLOOD FLOW

Cerebral Circulation
The cerebral circulation follows the same physiological principles of other circulatory beds such as the *Ohm's law*:

$$F = \frac{P_i - P_O}{R}$$

where

F = flow
P_i = input pressure
P_o = outflow pressure
R = resistance

The term "$P_i - P_o$" is referred as the cerebral perfusion pressure (CPP)

Cerebral Perfusion Pressure
The *cerebral perfusion pressure* (CPP) can be estimated by the following formula:

$$\textbf{CPP} = \text{MAP} - \text{ICP}$$

where

MAP = mean arterial pressure
ICP = intracranial pressure

Pressure–Volume Index
The *pressure–volume index* (PVI) can be calculated as:

$$\textbf{PVI} = \Delta V / [\log P_p / P_o]$$

where

P_p = Peak CSF pressure (increase after volume injection and decrease after volume withdrawal)

Cerebral Blood Flow
The *cerebral blood flow* (CQ) is normally 50 mL per 100 g/min and is determined by the *Hagen–Poiseuille equation* of flow through a tube:

$$\textbf{CQ} = \frac{(K \times \text{Pr}^4)}{(8L \times \eta)}$$

where

P = cerebral perfusion pressure (CPP)
r = arterial radius
η = blood viscosity
L = arterial length
K = constant

Local Cortical Cerebral Blood Flow
To assess the *local cortical cerebral blood flow* (CBF), the following formula can be employed:

$$\textbf{lCoCBF} = \varnothing \left(\frac{1}{\Delta V} - \frac{1}{\Delta V_0} \right)$$

where

ICoCBF = local cortical CBF
$\varnothing$ = constant value used as a scale factor
ΔV_0 = maximum temperature difference of zero blood flow
ΔV = actual temperature difference

Pulsatility Index
To assess flow velocity utilizing transcranial Doppler ultrasound, a resistance index such as the "*pulsatility index*" (PI) can be employed:

$$PI = \frac{\text{Systolic velocity} - \text{diastolic velocity}}{\text{Mean velocity}}$$

■ 3. BRAIN METABOLISM

Oxygen Availability to Neural Tissue
Oxygen availability to neural tissue (CDO_2) is reflected in the formula:

$$\mathbf{CDO_2} = CQ \times PaO_2$$

where

CQ = cerebral blood flow
PaO_2 = arterial oxygen concentration

Cerebral Metabolic Rate
The *cerebral metabolic rate* ($CMRO_2$) can be calculated as:

$$\mathbf{CMRO_2} = CBF \times AVDO_2$$

where

CBF = cerebral blood flow
$AVDO_2$ = arteriovenous oxygen content difference

Oxygen Extraction Ratio
The *oxygen extraction ratio* (OER) can be utilized to assess the brain metabolism:

$$\mathbf{OER} = SaO_2 - SjvO_2 / SaO_2$$

where

SaO_2 = arterial oxygen saturation
$SjvO_2$ = jugular venous oxygen saturation

$$\mathbf{OER} \times \mathbf{CaO_2} = CMRO_2 / CBF$$

where

$$CaO_2 = (Hb \times 1.39 \times SaO_2) + [0.003 \times PO_2 (mmHg)]$$

$$CMRO_2 = CBF \times (CaO_2 - CjvO_2)$$

Arterial-Jugular Venous Oxygen Content Difference
The *arterial-jugular venous oxygen content difference* (AjvDO$_2$) is calculated as:

$$AjvDO_2 = CMRO_2 / CBF$$

■ 4. MISCELLANEOUS

Muscle Strength Scale
The *Muscle Strength Scale* is used to evaluate muscle strength and is depicted in Table 7.7:

Table 7.7 The muscle strength scale

0	Total paralysis
1	Palpable or visible contraction
2	Active movement, full range of motion, gravity eliminated
3	Active movement, full range of motion, against gravity
4	Active movement, full range of motion, against gravity and provides some resistance
5	Active movement, full range of motion, against gravity and provides normal resistance
5˙	Muscle able to exert sufficient resistance to be considered normal if identifiable inhibiting factors were not present

Glasgow Coma Scale
The *Glasgow Coma Scale* (GSC) is commonly used in critically ill patients and is depicted in Table 7.8:

Table 7.8 Glasgow coma scale. Sum each response for the total score

Glasgow coma scale	
	Score
Eye opening	
Spontaneous	4
To verbal command	3
To pain	2
None	1
Best motor response	
Obeys verbal command	6
Localizes painful stimuli	5
Flexion withdrawal from painful stimuli	4
Decorticate (flexion) response to painful stimuli	3
Decerebrate (extension response to painful stimuli	2
None	1
Best verbal response	
Oriented conversation	5
Disoriented conversation	4
Inappropriate words	3
Incomprehensible sounds	2
None	1
	Total score 3–15/15

Apnea Test
The apnea test can be performed following the instructions depicted in Table 7.9:

Table 7.9 The Apnea test

1. Oxygenate with 100 % FiO_2 for 5–10 min before the test
2. Keep O_2 at 4–8 L/min flowing through the endotracheal tube while the patient is disconnected (if hypotension and/or dysrhythmias appear, immediately reconnect the ventilator. Stop this test. Consider other confirmatory tests)
3. Observe for spontaneous respirations
4. After 10 min have passed, obtain arterial blood gases. Patient is apneic if $PCO_2 \geq$ 60 Torr (mmhg) and there are no respiratory movements

Note: In patients with chronic obstructive pulmonary disease, the PaO$_2$ must be <50 Torr at the end of the apnea test

ABCD^2 Score
ABCD^2 Score is commonly used to assess a patient's stroke risk after a transient ischemic attack and is depicted in Table 7.10:

Table 7.10 ABCD^2 score

A (age)	1 point if age is >60 years old
B (blood pressure)	1 point if hypertensive at the acute evaluation
C (clinical features)	1 point for speech disturbance without weakness 2 points for unilateral weakness
D (symptom duration)	1 point for 10–59 min 2 points for ≥60 min
D (diabetes)	1 point if present

Low risk	0–3
Moderate risk	4–5
High risk	6–7

Dermatome Map
Dermatome Map is used to localize neurological lesions. It is depicted in Fig. 7.1.

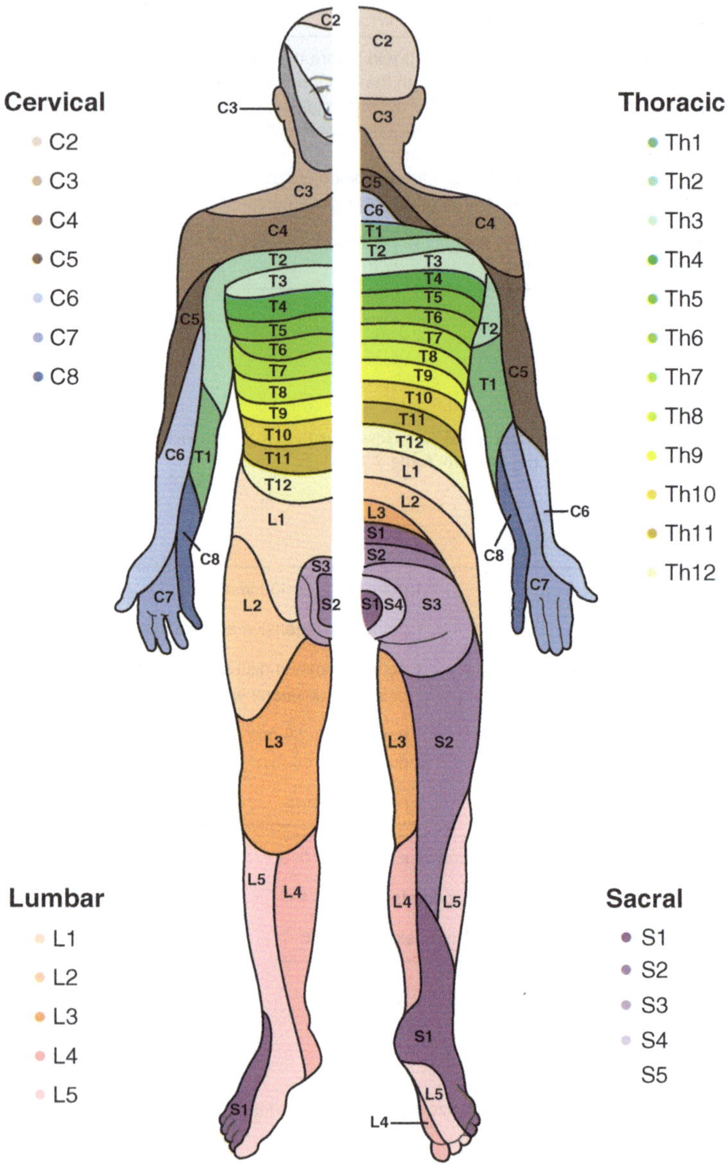

Cervical

- C2
- C3
- C4
- C5
- C6
- C7
- C8

Thoracic

- Th1
- Th2
- Th3
- Th4
- Th5
- Th6
- Th7
- Th8
- Th9
- Th10
- Th11
- Th12

Lumbar

- L1
- L2
- L3
- L4
- L5

Sacral

- S1
- S2
- S3
- S4
  S5

Fig. 7.1 Dermatomal distribution

American Spinal Injury Association

The *American Spinal Injury Association (ASIA) Impairment Scale* is used to classify and stratify spinal injuries (Table 7.11):

Table 7.11 The ASIA scale

A	Complete:	No motor or sensory function is preserved in the sacral segments S4–S5
B	Incomplete:	Sensory but not motor function is preserved below the neurological level and includes the sacral segments S4–S5
C	Incomplete:	Motor function is preserved below the neurological level and more than half of key muscles below the neurological level have a muscle grade <3
D	Incomplete:	Motor function is preserved below the neurological level, and at least half the key muscles below the neurological level have a muscle grade of ≥3
E	Normal:	Motor and sensory function are normal

CHA_2DS_2-*VASC Score*

The CHA_2DS_2-*VASC score* is used to estimate the risk of ischemic stroke in patients with nonrheumatic atrial fibrillation. It is depicted in Table 7.12:

Table 7.12 CHA$_2$DS$_2$-VASC score

C (chronic heart failure)	1 point
H (hypertension)	1 point
A (Age ≥ 75)	2 points
D (diabetes mellitus)	1 point
S (prior stroke)	2 points
V (vascular disease)	1 point
A (Age 65–74)	1 point
Sc (sex category)	1 point

Points	Risk (%/year)
0	0
1	1.3
2	2.2
3	3.2
4	4
5	6.7
6	9.8
7	9.6
8	6.7
9	15.2

Modified Rankin Scale
The *modified Rankin scale* is used to evaluate disability after a neurological event (Table 7.13):

Table 7.13 The modified Rankin scale

0	No symptoms at all
1	No significant disability despite symptoms; able to carry out all usual duties and activities
2	Slight disability; unable to carry out all previous activities, but able to look after own affairs without assistance
3	Moderate disability; requiring some help, but able to walk without assistance
4	Moderately severe disability; unable to walk without assistance and unable to attend to own bodily needs without assistance
5	Severe disability; bedridden, incontinent, and requiring constant nursing care and attention
6	Death

Ramsay Sedation Scale
The *Ramsay Sedation Scale* is useful to evaluate sedation levels in the Intensive Care Unit (Table 7.14):

Table 7.14 The Ramsay sedation scale

1	Anxious or restless or both
2	Cooperative, oriented, and calm
3	Responding to commands
4	Brisk response to stimulus
5	Sluggish response to stimulus
6	No response to stimulus

8

Nutrition Facts and Formulas

Adequate nutrition is paramount to optimize survival from critical illness. Many patients in intensive care units cannot or will not take adequate nutrition orally and, thus, supplementation of nutrients via alternative enteral or parenteral routes may be important. The following facts and formulas represent the information necessary for assessment and administration of nutritional support.

■ 1. NUTRITIONAL ASSESSMENT

Total Daily Energy

The *total daily energy* (TDE) requirements for a patient can be calculated using the following formula:

$$\textbf{TDE for men (kcal/day)} = (66.5 + 13.8W + 5H - 6.8A) \times (\text{Activity factor}) \times (\text{Injury factor})$$

$$\textbf{TDE for women (kcal / day)} = (655.10 + 9.6W + 1.9H - 4.7A) \times (\text{Activity factor}) \times (\text{Injury factor})$$

where
  W = weight (kg)
  H = height (cm)
  A = age (years)

The activity factor is derived as shown in Table 8.1:

J. Varon and R.E. Fromm Jr., *Acute and Critical Care Formulas and Laboratory Values*, DOI 10.1007/978-1-4614-7510-1_8,

Table 8.1 Activity factor

Confined to bed	1.2
Out of bed	1.3

Injury Factors
The *injury factors* can be estimated based on the information in Table 8.2:

Table 8.2 Injury factors

Surgery	
Minor	1.0–1.1
Major	1.1–1.3
Infection	
Mild	1.0–1.2
Moderate	1.2–1.4
Severe	1.4–1.8
Trauma	
Skeletal	1.2–1.4
Head injury with steroid therapy	1.6–1.8
Blunt	1.15–1.35
Burns (body surface area)	
Up to 20 %	1.0–1.5
20 % to 40 %	1.5–1.85
Over 40 %	1.85–1.95

Metabolic Rate
The *metabolic rate* (MR) can be calculated in patients with a pulmonary artery catheter as:

$$\mathbf{MR}\ (\mathbf{kcal\ /\ h}) = V\mathrm{O}_2(\mathrm{mL\ /\ min}) \times 60\ \mathrm{min/\ h} \times 1\ \mathrm{L\ /\ 1,000\ mL}$$
$$\times\ 4.83\ \mathrm{kcal\ /\ L} \times 24\ \mathrm{h\ /\ d}$$

where

$V\mathbf{O_2}\ (\mathbf{mL\ /\ min})$ = Cardiac output (L / min) × [arterial oxygen content $(\mathrm{CaO}_2, \mathrm{mL\ /\ L})$ − mixed venous oxygen content $(\mathrm{CmO}_2, \mathrm{mL\ /\ L})$]

Prognostic Nutritional Index

The *prognostic nutritional index* (PNI) allows for nutritional assessment of the critically ill patient and is calculated as:

$$\textbf{PNI (\%risk)} = 158\% - 16.6\,(\text{alb}) - 0.78\,(\text{TSF}) - 0.2\,(\text{tfn}) - 5.8\,(\text{DSH})$$

where

alb = serum albumin (g/dL)
TSF = triceps skin fold (mm)
tfn = serum transferrin (mg/dL)
DSH = delayed skin hypersensitivity (1 = anergy, 2 = reactive)

Probability of Survival

The *probability of survival* (POS) based on the nutritional status of a critically ill patient can be calculated as:

$$\textbf{POS} = 0.91\,(\text{alb}) - 1.0\,(\text{DSH}) - 1.44\,(\text{SEP}) + 0.98\,(\text{DIA}) - 1.09$$

where

alb = serum albumin (g/dL)
DSH = delayed skin hypersensitivity (1 = anergy, 2 = reactive)
SEP = sepsis (1 = no sepsis, 2 = sepsis)
DIA = diagnosis of cancer (1 = no cancer, 2 = cancer)

Index of Undernutrition

Another way to calculate the nutritional deficit is by utilizing the *index of undernutrition* (IOU) (see Table 8.3):

Table 8.3 Index of undernutrition

| | *Points* | | | | |
Assay	*0*	*5*	*10*	*15*	*20*
Albumin (g/dL)	>3.5	3.1–3.5	2.6–3.0	2.0–2.5	<2.0
Fat area (%)	>70	56–70	46–55	30–45	<30
Muscle area (%)	>80	76–80	61–75	40–60	<40
Transferrin (g/L)	>2.0	1.76–2.0	1.41–1.75	1.0–1.4	<40
Weight lost (%)	0	0–10	11–14	15–20	>20

Daily Protein Requirements
The calculation of *daily protein requirements* (PR) can be done utilizing the following formula:

$$\textbf{PR (g)} = (\text{Patient weight in kg}) \times (\text{PR for illness in g / kg})$$

Nonprotein Caloric Requirements
In order to determine the nonprotein caloric requirements (NCR):

$$\textbf{NCR} = (\text{Total required calories}) - (\text{Required protein calories})$$

Nitrogen Balance
The *nitrogen balance* (NB) reflects the status of the net protein use:

$$\textbf{NB} = (\text{Dietary protein} \times 0.16) - (\text{UUN} + 2\text{ g stool} + 2\text{ g skin})$$

where

UUN = urine urea nitrogen

In patients with renal failure, the increased blood urea pool and extrarenal urea losses must be accounted for:

$$\textbf{NB} = \text{Nitrogen in} - (\text{UUN} + 2\text{ g stool} + 2\text{ g skin} + \text{BUN change})$$

Catabolic Index
In addition to the above formulas, the *catabolic index* (CI) can be derived from the same variables:

$$\textbf{CI} = \text{UUN} - [(0.5 \times \text{Dietary protein} \times 0.16) + 3\text{ g}]$$

No nutritional stress results in a $CI \leq 0$, in moderate nutritional stress $CI < 5$, and in severe nutritional stress > 5.

Creatinine Height Index
Another index of the loss of lean tissue in malnourished patients is the *creatinine height index* (CHI) and can be calculated as:

$$\textbf{CHI} = \text{Measured creatinine / expected creatinine}$$

Body Mass Index
The *body mass index* (BMI) normalizes for height and allows comparisons among diverse populations:

$$\textbf{BMI} = \text{Body weight (kg) / (height)}^2 \text{ (m)}$$

Harris–Benedict Equation

The *Harris–Benedict equation* (HBE) is frequently utilized in assessment of the basal energy expenditure [BEE]:

$$\mathbf{HBE\ BEE} = 66 + [13.7 \times (5 \times H) - 6.8 \times A]\,\text{males}$$
$$= 665 + (9.6 \times W) + (1.7 \times H) - (4.7 \times A)\,\text{females}$$

where

W = weight (kg)
H = height (cm)
A = age (years)

■ 2. FUEL COMPOSITION

The body uses different sources of fuel. Table 8.4 depicts some of them:

Table 8.4 Normal fuel composition of the human body

Fuel	Amount (kg)	Calories (kcal)
Circulating fuels		
Glucose	0.020	80
Free fatty acids (plasma)	0.0003	3
Triglycerides (plasma)	0.003	30
Ketone bodies	0.0002	0.8
Amino acids	0.006	24
Total		137.8
Tissue		
Fat (adipose triglycerides)	12	110,000
Protein (muscle)	6	24,000
Glycogen (muscle)	0.4	1,600
Glycogen (liver)	0.08	320
Total		135,920

■ 3. OTHER FORMULAS

Body Surface Area
The *body surface area* (BSA) of a patient can be calculated as:

$$\mathbf{BSA}\,(\mathbf{m^2}) = \frac{(\text{Weight in kg})^{0.425} \times (\text{height in cm})^{0.725} \times 71.84}{10,000}$$

Ideal Body Weight
The *ideal body weight* (IBW) for height in males and females can be estimated based on Table 8.5:

Table 8.5 Ideal body weight in males and females

Height in cm	Males (weight in kg)	Females (weight in kg)
145	51.8	47.5
150	54.5	50.4
155	57.2	53.1
160	60.5	56.2
165	63.5	59.5
175	70.1	66.3
180	74.2	
185	78.1	

Percentage of Ideal Body Weight
The *percentage of ideal body weight* (%IBW) is calculated as:

$$\mathbf{\%IBW} = \frac{\text{Actual body weight}}{\text{IBW}} \times 100$$

where

W= actual body weight (kg)

9

Obstetrics and Gynecology Facts and Formulas

In most instances female patients in the ED and ICU are managed identically to male patients. The issues of pregnancy and medical conditions unique to women, of course, are an exception. The following tables and formulas should be useful to the practitioner caring for pregnant patients.

■ 1. HEMODYNAMICS

The hemodynamic changes that occur in pregnancy are depicted in Tables 9.1 and 9.2:

Table 9.1 Hemodynamic changes during pregnancy

Parameter	Change	Peak of changes
Cardiac output	Increases 30–50 %	28–32 weeks
Heart rate	Increases 10–15 %	32 weeks
Stroke volume	Increases 25–30 %	16–24 weeks
Blood volume		
Plasma	Increases 40–60 %	32 weeks
Red blood cells	Increase 25–33 %	30–32 weeks
Total body water	Increases 6–8 L	Term

(continued)

J. Varon and R.E. Fromm Jr., *Acute and Critical Care Formulas and Laboratory Values*, DOI 10.1007/978-1-4614-7510-1_9, © Springer Science+Business Media New York 2014

Table 9.1 (continued)

Parameter	Change	Peak of changes
Blood pressure		
Systemic	Decreases or not	
Diastolic	Decreases 10–15 mmHg	24–32 weeks
Oxygen consumption	Increases 20–30 %	Term
Systemic resistance	Decreases −20 %	16–34 weeks
Pulmonary resistance	Decreases −34 %	34 weeks
Pulmonary artery pressure	No change	
Myocardial function		
Chronotropism	Increases 10–20 %	28–32 weeks
Inotropism	Increases 25–30 %	16–24 weeks
Oxygen consumption	Increases 20–30 %	Term
Oxygen delivery	Increases 700–1,400 mL/min or not	Term

Table 9.2 Hemodynamic effects of labor and delivery

Parameter	Effect
Cardiac output	Increases with contractions
Blood volume	Increases
Heart rate	Variable
Peripheral resistance	No change
Systemic arterial pressure	Increases

The hemodynamic responses expected in response to position changes in the third trimester of pregnancy are depicted in Table 9.3:

Table 9.3 Hemodynamic changes in response to position change late in the third trimester of pregnancy

Hemodynamic parameter	Left lateral	Supine	Sitting	Standing
MAP (mmHg)	90 ± 6	90 ± 8	90 ± 8	91 ± 14
Cardiac output (L/min)	6.6 ± 1.4	6.0 ± 1.4[a]	6.2 ± 2.05	4 ± 2.0[a]
Pulse (bmp)	82 ± 10	84 ± 10	91 ± 11	107 ± 17[a]
Systemic vascular resistance (dynes × s/cm^5)	1,210 ± 266	1,437 ± 338	1,217 ± 254	1,319 ± 394
Pulmonary vascular resistance (dynes × s/cm^5)	76 ± 16	101 ± 45	102 ± 35	117 ± 35[a]
Pulmonary capillary wedge pressure (mmHg)	8 ± 2	6 ± 3	4 ± 4	4 ± 2
Central venous pressure (mmHg)	4 ± 3	3 ± 2	1 ± 1	1 ± 2
Left ventricular stroke work index (gm-m/m²/beat)	43 ± 9	40 ± 9	44 ± 5	34 ± 7[a]

[a]Pulse <0.05, compared with left lateral position

Uterine Oxygen Consumption
Uterine oxygen consumption can be calculated by the following formula:

$$\textbf{O}_2 \textbf{ Uptake by Gravid Uterus} = (A - V) \times F$$

where

    A = material arterial blood oxygen content
    V = uterine venous blood oxygen content
    F = uterine blood flow

Oxygen Saturation of the Uterine Venous Blood
The *oxygen saturation of the uterine venous blood* flow (Sv) is another important parameter to follow and is calculated as:

$$Sv + SaO_2 - VO_2(O_2Cap)$$

where

SaO$_2$ = maternal oxygen saturation
VO_2 = oxygen consumption rate
Sv = uterine blood flow
O$_2$ Cap = oxygen capacity of maternal blood

■ 2. PULMONARY

The changes expected during pregnancy in pulmonary function are depicted in Table 9.4:

Table 9.4 Lung volumes and capacities in pregnancy

	Definition	Change in pregnancy
Respiratory rate (RR)	Number of breaths per minute	Unchanged
Vital capacity (VC)	Maximum amount of air that can be forcibly expired after a maximum inspiration (IC + ERV)	Unchanged
Inspiratory capacity (IC)	Maximum amount of air that can be inspired from resting expiratory level (TV + IRV)	Increased 5 %
Tidal volume (VT)	Amount of air inspired and expired with normal breath	Increased 30–40 %
Inspiratory reserve volume (IRV)	Maximum amount of air that can be inspired at the end of normal inspiration	Unchanged
Functional residual capacity (FRC)	Amount of air in lungs at resting expiratory level (ERV + RV)	Decreased 20 %
Expiratory reserve volume (ERV)	Maximum amount of air that can be expired from resting expiratory level	Decreased 20 %
Residual volume (RV)	Amount of air in lungs after maximum expiration	Decreased 20 %
Total lung capacity (TLC)	Total amount of air in lungs at maximal inspiration (VC + RV)	Decreased 5 %

■ 3. OTHER FORMULAS

Naegele's Rule
If the last menstrual period (LMP) is known, the probable delivery date (DD) can be approximated utilizing *Naegele's rule*:

$$\textbf{DD} = \text{First day of LMP} + 7 \text{ days-3 months}$$

Weight Gain
The approximate *weight gain* by a pregnant woman can be calculated after the second trimester as:

$$\textbf{WG} = 225 \text{ g} \times \text{weeks of gestation}$$

Intraperitoneal Fetal Transfusion
Occasionally there is a need for *intraperitoneal fetal transfusion* in a gravid patient. The following formula is used to calculate the volume of red blood cells (RBC) to be injected into the fetal peritoneal cavity (IPT volume):

$$\textbf{IPT volume} = (\text{weeks' gestation} - 20) \times 10 \text{ mL}$$

Bowman's Formula
To determine the concentration of donor hemoglobin present in the fetus at any time following an intrauterine transfusion, *Bowman's formula* is applied:

$$\textbf{Hb concentration (g/dL)} = \frac{0.55 \times a}{85 \times b} \times \frac{120 - c}{120}$$

where

0.55 = fraction of transfused RBC in the fetal circulation
a = amount of donor RBC transfused (g)
b = fetal weight (kg)
c = interval (days) from the time of transfusion to the time of calculation
85 = estimation of blood volume (mL/kg) in the fetus
120 = life span of donor RBC

Placental Transfer of Drugs
The *placental transfer of drugs* can be calculated as:

$$\textbf{Q / t} = \frac{KA(C_m - C_f)}{D}$$

where

Q/t = rate of diffusion
K = diffusion constant
A = surface area available for exchange
C_m = concentration of free drug in maternal blood
C_f = concentration of free drug in fetal blood
D = thickness of diffusion barrier

10

Oncology Facts and Formulas

Cancer patients comprise a large portion of those needing acute and critical care services. These patients may require critical care on a short-term basis for the complications of the underlying malignancy or for aggressive antineoplastic therapy. The following formulas and facts will aid the clinician in the diagnosis and management of these patients.

■ 1. BASIC ONCOLOGY FORMULAS

Although not clinically useful, these formulas allow a better understanding of the oncogenesis process, its complications, and response to therapy.

Growth Factor
The rapidly proliferating component of human tumors is known as the *growth factor* (GF) and is calculated as:

$$\mathbf{GF} = \frac{\text{Observed fraction of cells in } S}{\text{Expected fraction of cells in } S}$$

where

S = part of cell cycle where DNA synthesis occurs predominantly

Thymidine Labeling Index
The fraction of cells in "S" phase can be assessed by titrated thymidine labeling and autoradiography. The fraction of labeled cells is known as the *thymidine labeling index* (TLI):

$$\mathbf{TLI} = \frac{\text{Number of labeled cells}}{\text{Total number of cells}}$$

J. Varon and R.E. Fromm Jr., *Acute and Critical Care Formulas and Laboratory Values*, DOI 10.1007/978-1-4614-7510-1_10,
© Springer Science+Business Media New York 2014

■ 2. NUTRITION IN CANCER

Also refer to Chap. 8.

Percent Weight Change
Cancer patients are frequently malnourished and require close nutritional monitoring. To assess the amount of weight loss (*percent weight change*) that these patients have the following formula is utilized:

$$\textbf{Percent weight change} = \frac{(\text{Usual weight} - \text{Actual weight})}{(\text{Usual weight})} \times 100$$

The evaluation of weight change bases on the percent weight change formula is depicted in Table 10.1:

Table 10.1 Evaluation of weight change based on the percent weight change formula

	Significant weight loss (%)	Severe weight loss (%)
7 days	1–2	>2
1 month	5	>5
3 months	7.5	>7.5
6 months	10	>10
Unlimited time period	10–20	>20

Nitrogen Balance
A useful formula in the nutritional assessment of these patients relates to the *nitrogen balance*:

$$\textbf{Nitrogen balance} = \frac{\text{Protein intake (g)}}{6.25} - (24\text{-h urine urea nitrogen} + 4\text{ g})$$

Catabolic Index
The *catabolic index* (ID) aids in the identification of the amount of "nutritional stress" that these patients have:

$$\textbf{CI} = \text{Urinary urea nitrogen} - [0.5 \times \text{protein intake} \times 0.16) + 3\text{ g}]$$

The interpretation of the Catabolic index is depicted in Table 10.2:

Table 10.2 Interpretation of the catabolic index

Catabolic index	Interpretation
<0	No significant stress
0–5	Moderate stress
>5	Severe stress

Arm Muscle Circumference

The *arm muscle circumference* (AMC) is another sensitive measure of protein nutritional status in cancer patients also called mid-upper arm muscle circumference (MUAMC):

$$\textbf{MUAMC (cm)} = \text{arm circumference (cm)} - (3.14 \times \text{TSF [mmL]}) / 10$$

where

TSF = triceps skinfold measurement

■ 3. OTHER FACTS

The cerebrospinal fluid (CSF) findings in patients with *carcinomatous meningitis* are depicted in Table 10.3:

Table 10.3 CSF findings in patients with carcinomatous meningitis

Parameter	Percent of abnormal patients	Range
Opening pressure	50	60–450
WBC count	52	0–1,800
Glucose	30–38	0–244
Protein	30–81	24–2,485
Cytology	41–70	24–2,485

Pericardial Tamponade
Pericardial tamponade represents one of the complications that can occur in cancer patients. Its hemodynamic interpretation is depicted in Table 10.4:

Table 10.4 Hemodynamic parameters of pericardial tamponade and pericardial constriction

	Pericardial tamponade	*Pericardial constriction*
Right atrial pressure	$\geq$15 mmHg	$\geq$15 mmHg usually with prominent "*y*" trough
Left atrial pressure	Equals right atrial pressure	Equals right atrial pressure
Right ventricular pressure	No diastolic dip	Consistent early
Right ventricular diastolic pressure	$\leq$1/3 systolic blood pressure	$\geq$1/3 systolic right ventricular pressure
Pulmonary artery pressure	Systolic pulmonary artery pressure often $\leq$40 mmHg	Systolic pulmonary artery pressure <40 mmHg
Cardiac output	Decreased	Usually normal with normal arteriovenous difference
Respiratory variation in pressure	Usually present	Absent
Diastolic pressures	Equal	Equal

Body Surface Area
The *body surface area* (BSA) of a patient can be calculated as:

$$\textbf{BSA}\,(\textbf{m}^2) = ([\text{Height (cm)} \times \text{Weight (kg)}]\,/\,3,600)^{1/2}$$

11

Pediatric Facts, Formulas, and Laboratory Values

In no other area of critical care are formulas as important as in pediatrics. The large variation in patient size requires that simple rules of thumb be available to the critical care practitioner.

■ 1. AIRWAYS

Selecting the proper *size* (internal diameter [I.D.]) endotracheal tube (ETT) in children is important.

Cole Formula
The *Cole formula* is commonly utilized:

$$\textbf{Tube size (mm ID)} = \frac{\text{Age (year)}}{4} + 4$$

or

$$\textbf{Tube size (mm ID)} = \frac{16 + \text{Age (year)}}{4}$$

ETT in Newborns
The estimation of the *ETT in newborns* can be accomplished by utilizing the following formula:

$$\textbf{Tubesize (mm ID)} = \frac{\text{Postconceptual age in weeks}}{10}$$

J. Varon and R.E. Fromm Jr., *Acute and Critical Care Formulas and Laboratory Values*, DOI 10.1007/978-1-4614-7510-1_11, © Springer Science+Business Media New York 2014

Distance for Insertion
The proper *distance for insertion* of endotracheal tubes in children older than 2 years can be approximated by utilizing the following formulas:

$$\textbf{Distance (cm)} = \frac{\text{Age (yr)}}{2} + 12$$

or

$$\textbf{Depth of insertion} = \text{ETT ID} \times 3$$

■ **2. HEMODYNAMICS**

Median Systolic Blood Pressure
Normal blood pressure values vary according to age. The *median systolic blood pressure* (SBP) for children than 1 year is approximated by the following formula:

$$\textbf{SBP} = 90 \text{ mmHg} + (2 \times \text{age in years})$$

Lower Limit of the SBP
The *lower limit* of the SBP (SBP$_{LL}$) can be estimated as:

$$\textbf{SBP}_{LL} = 70 \text{ mmHg} + (2 \times \text{age in years})$$

Diastolic Blood Pressure
The *diastolic blood pressure* (DBP) calculation is:

$$\textbf{DBP} = 2/3 \times \text{systolic blood pressure}$$

Normal Heart Rate
The *normal heart rate* (HR) varies according to age. Table 11.1 depicts normal heart rate at different age groups:

Table 11.1 Heart rate at different age intervals

Age	Heart rate/min
0–1 month	100–180 (150)
2–3 months	110–180 (120)
4–12 months	100–180 (150)
1–3 years	100–180 (130)
4–5 years	60–150 (100)
6–8 years	60–130 (100)
9–11 years	50–110 (80)
12–16 years	50–100 (75)
>16 years	50–90 (70)

■ 3. INTRAVENOUS CANNULATION

The equipment necessary varies according to the age and weight of the pediatric critical care patient.

Over-the-Needle Catheters
Table 11.2 is a comparison table of different gauge for *over-the-needle catheters* for pediatric patients:

Table 11.2 Catheter gauge for over-the-needle cannulation in pediatric critically ill patients

Age (years)	Weight (kg)	Gauge
<1	<10	20, 22, 24
1–12	10–40	16, 18, 20
>12	>40	14, 16, 18

Umbilical Vein Catheterization
For *umbilical vein catheterization* is important to have a precise catheter length to place this catheter in the inferior vena cava. The following formula can be used for this estimation:

$$\text{UV catheter length (cm)} = 0.5 \times \text{UA catheter length (cm)} + 1$$

Umbilical Artery Catheterization
For *umbilical artery catheterization*:

$$\text{UA catheter length (cm)} = 3 \times \text{birth weight in kg} + 9$$

■ 4. NUTRITION

Estimated Body Weight
Estimating the *body weight* in children can be done utilizing the following formula:

$$\text{Estimated body weight (kg)} = (\text{Age in years} \times 2) + 8$$

Body Mass Index
For *Body mass index*:

$$\text{BMI} = \text{Weight in kg} / \text{Height in meters}^2$$

Mosteller Formula
For *Body surface area (Mosteller formula)*:

$$\text{BSA} = ([\text{Height (cm)} \times \text{Weight (kg)}] / 3{,}600)^{1/2}$$

Basal Metabolic Rate

The *energy needs* (basal metabolic rate or BMR) for a pediatric patient can be calculated using the following formulas:

$$\textbf{BMR males} = 66 + (13.7 \times W) + (5.0 \times H) - (6.8 \times A)$$

$$\textbf{BMR females} = 665 + (9.56 \times Wt) + 1.85 \times H - (4.7 \times A)$$

where

W = weight in kilograms
H = height in centimeters
A = age in years

Catabolic Index

To evaluate the *nutritional stress* of the pediatric patient in the intensive care unit, the catabolic index (CI) can be used:

$$\textbf{CI} = UUN - (0.5 \times N_{in} \times 0.16 + 3)$$

where

UUN = 24-h urine urea nitrogen in g
N_{in} = 24-h nitrogen intake in g

For additional formulas, please refer to Chap. 8.

■ **5. WATER REQUIREMENTS**

Water requirements for children vary according to age and weight of child (see Table 11.3):

Table 11.3 Maintenance fluid requirements of children

Weight	Maintenance fluids (mL/day)	Maintenance fluid (mL/h)
<10 kg	100 mL/kg	4 mL/kg
11–20 kg	1,000 mL + 50 mL/kg/24 h for each kg over 10 kg	40 mL + mL/kg
20–80 kg	1,500 mL + 20 mL/kg/24 h for each kg over 20 kg	60 mL + 1 mL/kg

■ 6. CATION REQUIREMENTS

Daily major *cation requirements* in the youngsters can be summarized as follows:

$$Na^+ = 3 \text{ mEq / kg / 24 h (maximum 80 mEq / 24 h)}$$

$$K^+ = 2 \text{ mEq / kg / 24 h (maximum 40 mEq / 24 h)}$$

■ 7. URINARY LOSSES

Urinary losses (UL) reflect the solute load, excretion, and urine concentration:

$$UL = 60 \text{ mL / kg / 24 h}$$

■ 8. FECAL LOSSES

In general, *fecal losses* (FL) are small in young children and insignificant in older children:

$$FL = 10 \text{ mL / kg / 24 h}$$

■ 9. INSENSIBLE LOSSES

Insensible losses (IL) mostly occur through skin and respiratory tract:

$$IL = 30 \text{ mL / kg / 24 h}$$

Fever increases IL by 7 mL/kg/24 h for each degree rise in temperature above 37.2 °C (99 °F).

■ 10. HEMATOLOGICAL FORMULAS

Required Packed Cell Volume
In order to estimate the *required packed cell volume*, use the formula:

$$\textbf{Vol. of cells (mL)} = \frac{\text{Estimated blood volume (mL)} \times \text{Desired Hct change}}{\text{Hct of PRBC}}$$

Rapid Correction of the Hemoglobin
In patients with severe anemia, *rapid correction of the hemoglobin* can be achieved utilizing the formula:

$$\textbf{Volume (mL)} = \frac{\text{Blood volume (mL)} \times \text{Desired Hb rise}}{22 \text{ g} / \text{dL} - \text{HbR}}$$

where

$$\textbf{HbR} = \frac{\text{Desired Hb} - \text{Initial Hb}}{2}$$

Exchange Transfusion
In pediatric patients undergoing *exchange transfusion*, the following formula can be applied:

$$\textbf{V} = \frac{(\text{Hct}_f - \text{Hct}_i) \times \text{Body weight (kg)} \times 70 \text{ mL} / \text{kg}}{\text{Hct}_i}$$

where

V = volume to be exchanged
Hct_f = final hematocrit
Hct_i = initial hematocrit

■ 11. OTHER FORMULAS

Stool Osmotic Gap
Occasionally it is necessary to calculate the *stool osmotic gap* (SOG) to determine the type of diarrhea (i.e., secretory, malabsorption, etc.). The stool osmotic gap can be calculated with the formula:

$$\textbf{SOG} = 280 - 2 \times (\text{Na}^+ + \text{K}^+)$$

Glucose Infusion in Newborns
The formula utilized to calculate the rate of *glucose infusion in newborns* is:

$$\textbf{Glucose infusion (mg / kg / min glucose)} = \frac{\%\text{Glucose} \times \text{mL} / \text{kg} / \text{d}}{144}$$

or

$$\textbf{Glucose infusion (mg / kg / min glucose)} = \frac{\%\text{Glucose} \times \text{mL} / \text{kg} / \text{h}}{6 \times \text{body weight (kg)}}$$

■ 12. SELECTED PEDIATRIC LABORATORY VALUES

Blood = (B), Serum = (S), Plasma = (P), Urine = (U), Red blood cells = (RBC)

Neonatal Acid-Base Measurement (B)

pH: 7.35–7.45
PaO_2: 50–70 mmHg (8.66–10.13 kPa)
$PaCO_2$: 35–45 mmHg (4.8–5.07 kPa)
Base excess: ±4 mEq/L

Acid Phosphatase (S, P)

Vales using p-nitrophenyl phosphate buffered with citrate.
Newborns: 7.4–19.4 IU/L at 37 °C
2–13 years: 6.4–15.2 IU/L at 37 °C
Adult males: 0.5–11 IU/L at 37 °C
Adult females: 0.2–9.5 IU/L at 37 °C

Alanine Aminotransferase (ALAT, ALT, SGPT) (S)

Newborns: 13–45 U/L
Adult males: 10–40 U/L
Adult females: 4–35+ U/L

Aldolase (S)

Newborns: 17.5–47.8 UI/L at 37 °C
Children: 8.8–23.9 IU/L at 37 °C
Adults: 4.4–12 IU/L at 37 °C

Ammonia (P)

Newborns: 90–150 μg/dL (53–88 μmol/L); higher in premature and jaundiced
infants; thereafter 0–60 μg/dL (0–35 μmol/L) when blood is drawn with proper
precautions.

Amylase

0–30 days: 0–6 U/L
31–182 days: 1–17 U/L
183–365 days: 6–44 U/L
1–3 years: 8–79 U/L
4–17 years: 21–110 U/L
> or 18 years: 26–102 U/L

Aspartate Aminotransferase (ASAT, AST, SGOT) (S)

Males

0–11 months: not established
1–13 years: 8–60 U/L
> or =14 years: 8–48 U/L

Females

0–11 months: not established
1–13 years: 8–50 U/L
≥14 years: 8–43 U/L

Bicarbonate Serum

Males

12–24 months: 17–25 mmol/L
3 years: 18–26 mmol/L
4–5 years: 19–27 mmol/L
6–7 years: 20–28 mmol/L
8–17 years: 21–29 mmol/L
≥18 years: 22–29 mmol/L

Females

1–3 years: 18–25 mmol/L
4–5 years: 19–26 mmol/L
6–7 years: 20–27 mmol/L
8–9 years: 21–28 mmol/L
≥ 10 years: 22–29 mmol/L

Bilirubin Serum

Direct

≥12 months: 0.0–0.3 mg/dL

Reference values have not been established for patients that are less than 12 months of age.

Total

Males

12 months: 0.1–0.9 mg/dL
≥ 24 months: 0.1–1.0 mg/dL

Reference values have not been established for patients that are less than 12 months of age.

Females

1–11 years: 0.1–0.9 mg/dL
≥12 years: 0.1–1.0 mg/dL

Bleeding Time (Simplate)

2–9 min

Blood Volume

Premature infants: 98 mL/kg
At 1 year: 86 mL/kg (range, 69–112 mL/kg)
Older children: 70 mL/kg (range, 51–86 mL/kg)

Calcium (S)

Males

1–14 years: 9.6–10.6 mg/dL
15–16 years: 9.5–10.5 mg/dL
17–18 years: 9.5–10.4 mg/dL
19–21 years: 9.3–10.3 mg/dL
≥22 years: 8.9–10.1 mg/dL

Females

1–11 years: 9.6–10.6 mg/dL
12–14 years: 9.5–10.4 mg/dL
15–18 years: 9.1–10.3 mg/dL
≥19 years: 8.9–10.1 mg/dL

Carbon Dioxide Total (S, P)

Umbilical cord blood: 15–20.2 mmol/L
Children: 18–27 mmol/L
Adults: 24–35 mmol/L

Carboxyhemoglobin (B)

5 % of total hemoglobin

Chloride (S, P)

1–17 years: 102–112 mmol/L
≥18 years: 100–108 mmol/L

Cholesterol, Total (S, P) (see Table 11.4)

Values in mg/dL (mmol/L)

Table 11.4 Cholesterol values in childhood

Age group (years)	Value for males	Values for females
6–7	115–197 (2.97–5.09)	126–199 (3.25–5.14)
8–9	112–199 (2.89–5.14)	124–208 (3.20–5.37)
10–11	108–220 (2.79–5.68)	115–208 (2.97–5.37)
12–13	117–202 (3.02–5.21)	114–207 (2.94–5.34)
14–15	103–207 (2.66–5.34)	102–208 (2.63–5.37)
16–17	107–198 (92.76–5.11)	106–213 (2.73–5.50)

Cortisol (S,P)

A.M.

<16 years: not established
≥16 years: 5–25 mcg/dL

P.M.

<16 years: not established
≥16 years: 2–14 mcg/dL

Creatine Kinase Serum

Males

6–11 years: 150–499 U/L
12–17 years: 94–499 U/L
> or 18 years: 52–336 U/L

Females

6–7 years: 134–391 U/L
8–14 years: 91–391 U/L
15–17 years: 53–269 U/L
> or 18 years: 38–176 U/L

Creatinine (S,P) (see Table 11.5)

Values in mg/dL (µmol/L)

Table 11.5 Normal creatinine values in childhood

Age group	Values for males	Values for females
Newborns (1–3 days)[a]	0.2–1.0 (17.7–88.4)	0.2–1.0 (17.7–88.4)
1 year	0.2–0.6 (17.7–53.0)	0.2–0.5 (17.7–44.2)
2–3 years	0.2–0.7 (17.7–61.9)	0.3–0.6 (26.5–53.0)
4–7 years	0.2–0.8 (17.7–70.7)	0.2–0.7 (17.7–61.9)
8–10 years	0.3–0.9 (26.5–79.6)	0.3–0.8 (26.5–70.7)
11–12 years	0.3–1.0 (26.5–88.4)	0.3–0.9 (26.5–79.6)
13–17 years	0.3–1.2 (26.5–106.1)	0.3–1.1 (26.5–97.2)

[a]Values may be higher in premature newborns

Creatinine Clearance

Newborns (1–6 days): 5–50 mL/min/1.73 m^2 (mean, 18 mL/min/1.73 m^2).
Newborns (>6 days): 15–90 mL/min/1.73 m^2 (mean 36 mL/min/1.73 m^2)
Adult males: 85–125 mL/min/1.73 m^2
Adult females: 75–115 mL/min/1.73 m^2

Fibrinogen (P)

Males: 200–375 mg/dL
Females: 200–430 mg/dL

Glomerular Filtration Rate

Newborns: About 50 % of values for older children and adults
Older children and adults: 75–165 mL/min/1.73 m^2 (levels reached by about 6 months)

Haptoglobin (S)

50–150 mg/dL has hemoglobin–binding capacity.

Hematocrit (B)

At birth: 44–64 %
14–90 days: 35–49 %
6 months–1 year: 30–40 %
4–10 years: 31–43 %

Lactate (B)

Venous blood: 5–18 mg/dL (0.5–2 mmol/L)
Arterial blood: 3–7 mg/dL (0.3–0.8 mmol/L)

Lactate Dehydrogenase (LDH) (S,P)

Newborns (1–3 days): 40–348 IU/L at 37 °C
1 month–5 years: 150–360 IU/L at 37 °C
5–8 years: 150–300 IU/L at 37 °C
8–12 years: 130–300 IU/L at 37 °C
12–14 years: 130–280 IU/L at 37 °C
14–16 years: 130–230 IU/L at 37 °C
Adult males: 70–178 IU/L at 37 °C
Adult females: 42–166 IU/L at 37 °C

Lactate Dehydrogenase Isoenzymes (S)

LDH_1 (heart): 24–34 %
LDH_2 (heart, red blood cells): 35–45 %
LDH_3 (muscle): 15–25 %
LDH_4 (liver [trace], muscle) 4–10 %
LDH_5 (liver, muscle): 1–9 %

Lead (B)

<10 µg/dL (<0.48 µmol/L)

Lipase (S,P)

20–136 IU/L based on 4-h incubation

Magnesium Serum

0–2 years: 1.6–2.7 mg/dL
3–5 years: 1.6–2.6 mg/dL
6–8 years: 1.6–2.5 mg/dL
9–11 years: 1.6–2.4 mg/dL
12–17 years: 1.6–2.3 mg/dL
>17 years: 1.7–2.3 mg/dL

Magnesium (RBC)

3.92–5.28 mEq/L (1.96–2.64 mmol/L)

Manganese (S)

Newborns: 2.4–9.6 µg/dL (0.44–1.75 µmol/L)
Adults: 1.4–2 µg/dL (0.15–0.38 µmol/L)

Methemoglobin and Sulfhemoglobin, Blood

Methemoglobin

0–11 months: not established
≥1 year: 0.0–1.5 % of total hemoglobin

Sulfhemoglobin

0–11 months: not established
≥1 year: 0.0–0.4 % of total hemoglobin

Osmolality

Feces

220–280 mOsm/kg

Urine

0–11 months: 50–750 mOsm/kg
≥12 months: 150–1,150 mOsm/kg

Oxygen Capacity (B)

1.34 mL/g of hemoglobin

Oxygen Saturation [Venous] (B)

Newborns: 30–80 % (0.3–0.8 mol/mol of venous blood)
Thereafter: 65–85 % (0.65–0.85 mol/mol of venous blood)

Partial Thromboplastin Time (P)

Children: 42–54 s

Phosphorus Inorganic (S,P)

Premature infants:

At birth: 5.6–8 mg/dL (1.81–2.58 mmol/L)
6–10 days: 6.1–11.7 mg/dL (1.97–3.78 mmol/L)
20–25 days: 6.6–9.4 mg/dL (2.13–3.04 mmol/L)

Full-term infants:

At birth: 5–7.8 mg/dL (1.61–2.52 mmol/L)
3 days: 5.8–9 mg/dL (1.87–2.91 mmol/L)
6–12 days: 4.9–8.9 mg/dL (1.58–2.87 mmol/L)

Children:

1 year: 3.8–6.2 mg/dL (1.23–2 mmol/L)
10 years: 3.6–5.6 mg/dL (1.16–1.81 mmol/L)

Potassium (S,P)

Premature infants: 4.5–7.2 mmol/L
Full-term infants: 3.7–5.2 mmol/L
Children: 3.5–5.8 mmol/L
Adults: 3.5–5.5 mmol/L

Potassium (RBC)

Children: 87.2–97.6 mmol/L

Prothrombin Time (P)

Children: 11–15 s

Sedimentation Rate (B)

<2 years: 1–5 mm/h
>2 years: 1–8 mm/h

Sodium (S,P)

Children and adults: 135–148 mmol/L

Thrombin Time (P)

Children: 12–16 s

Triglyceride (S,P) (see Table 11.6)

Fasting (>12 h) values in mg/mL (mmol/L):

Table 11.6 Fasting triglyceride values in childhood

Age group (years)	Values for males	Values for females
6–7	32–79 (0.36–0.89)	24–128 (0.27–1.44)
8–9	28–105 (0.31–1.18	34–115 (0.38–1.29)
10–11	30–115 (0.33–1.29)	39–131 (0.44–1.48)
12–13	33–112 (0.37–1.26)	36–125 (0.40–1.41)
14–15	35–136 (0.39–1.53)	36–122 (0.40–1.37)
16–17	38–167 (0.42–1.88)	34–136 (0.38–1.53)

Urea Nitrogen (S,P)

1–2 years: 5–15 mg/dL (1.8–5.4 mmol/L)
Thereafter: 10–20 mg/dL (3.5–7.1 mmol/L)

Uric Acid (S,P)

Males:

0–14 years: 2–7 mg/dL (119–416 μmol/L)
>14 years: 3–8 mg/dL (178–476 μmol/L)

Females:

0–14 years: 2–7 mg/dL (119–416 μmol/L)
>14 years: 2–7 mg/dL (119–416 μmol/L)

Volume (B)

Premature infants: 98 mL/kg (mean)
Full-term infants: 75–100 mL/kg
1 year: 69–112 mL/kg (mean, 86 mL/kg)
Older children: 51–86 mL/kg (mean, 70 mL/kg)

Volume (P)

Full-term neonates: 39–77 mL/kg
Infants: 40–50 mL/kg
Older children: 30–54 mL/kg

Water (B,S,RBC)

Whole blood: 79–81 g/dL
Serum: 91–92 g/dL

12

Pulmonary Facts and Formulas

Pulmonary disorders are among the most common causes of admission to an intensive care unit and frequently seen in acute care medicine. The following formulas and facts are presented to aid in the diagnosis and management of patients presenting to the emergency department and the intensive care unit (ICU) with pulmonary conditions. Some of the formulas are not useful in the clinical area; however, their understanding is of paramount importance in understanding the normal and abnormal pulmonary physiology and therefore cannot be excluded from this chapter.

■ 1. LUNG VOLUMES

Normal values for pulmonary volumes and capacities in humans are depicted in Table 12.1:

Table 12.1 Normal values for lung volumes in upright subjects

Volume or capacity	Approximate value in upright subjects (L)
Total lung capacity (TLC)	6
Vital capacity (VC)	4.5
Residual volume (RV)	1.2
Inspiratory capacity (I_c)	3
Functional residual capacity (FRC)	3
Inspiratory reserve volume (IRV)	2.5
Expiratory reserve volume (ERV)	1.1
Tidal volume (V_T)	0.5

J. Varon and R.E. Fromm Jr., *Acute and Critical Care Formulas and Laboratory Values*, DOI 10.1007/978-1-4614-7510-1_12, © Springer Science+Business Media New York 2014

Vital Capacity
The *vital capacity* (VC) is calculated as:

$$\mathbf{VC} = IRV + ERV + V_T$$

Residual Volume
The *residual volume* (RV) is calculated as the difference between the functional residual capacity (FRC) and the expiratory reserve volume (ERV):

$$\mathbf{RV} = FRC - EV$$

Alternatively, if the total lung capacity (TLC) and vital capacity (VC) are known, the following formula can be utilized:

$$\mathbf{RV} = TLC - VC$$

Equilibration Technique
The oldest method to measure *FRC* is the *equilibration technique* utilizing the following formula:

$$\mathbf{FRC} = [(C_1 \times V_1) / C_2] - V_1$$

where

C_1 = known concentration of a test gas in the spirometer
V_1 = volume of gas in the spirometer
C_2 = fractional value of the gas after the subject breathes in the spirometer until the concentration of the test gas equals that in the spirometer

Nitrogen Washout Procedure
Another way to measure *FRC* is by utilizing the *nitrogen washout procedure* and the following formula:

$$\mathbf{FRC} = (V_B \times C_B) / C_X$$

where

V_B = amount of exhaled nitrogen volume in the bag
C_B = fractional concentration of nitrogen in the bag
C_X = subject initial fractional concentration of nitrogen (0.80)

Plethysmography
Alternatively, FRC can be calculated using body plethysmography as:

$$\mathbf{FRC} = (\Delta V / \Delta P)(P_B + \Delta P)$$

where

ΔV = change in volume
ΔP = change in pressure
P_B = atmospheric pressure minus water vapor pressure (PH_2O)

Tidal Volume
The *tidal volume* (V_T) is the sum of the dead space volume (V_D) and the alveolar volume (V_A):

$$\mathbf{V_T} = V_D + V_A$$

Dead Space Volume
The average *dead space volume* (V_D) is estimated as 1 mL/lb body weight. For an average 70-kg man:

$$\mathbf{V_D} = 70 \times 2.2 \times 1 = 154 \text{ mL}$$

■ **2. PULMONARY VENTILATION**

Minute Ventilation
The easiest way of estimating *minute ventilation* (V_E) is by using the following formula:

$$\mathbf{V_E} = V_T \times \text{RR} = \text{mL} / \min$$

where

V_T = tidal volume and RR is the respiratory rate

Minute ventilation is also the sum of dead space (V_D) and alveolar ventilation (V_A):

$$\mathbf{V_E} = V_A + V_D$$

Alveolar Ventilation
The *alveolar ventilation* (V_A) can be calculated as:

$$\mathbf{V_A} = (V_T - V_D) \times N$$

where

N = frequency of breathing in breaths per minute
V_D = dead space ventilation

Production of CO_2
An alternative method requires knowledge of the CO_2 production by the patient. The *production of CO_2* (VCO_2) can be calculated as:

$$\mathbf{VCO_2} = V_A \times F_A CO_2$$

where

$F_A CO_2$ = fractional concentration of CO_2 in the alveolar gas

$$\mathbf{V_A} = VCO_2 / F_A CO_2$$

Dead Space Ventilation
Dead space ventilation (V_D) can be calculated if the minute ventilation (V_E) is known:

$$\mathbf{V_D} = V_E ([PaCO_2 - P_E CO_2]) / PaCO_2$$

Partial Pressure of Alveolar CO_2
The *partial pressure of alveolar CO_2* ($P_A CO_2$) is more convenient for these calculations and for practical purposes:

$$\mathbf{P_A CO_2} = F_A CO_2 \times (P_B - 47)$$

Arterial CO_2
In normal lungs, the *arterial CO_2* ($PaCO_2$) approximates the $P_A CO_2$. Therefore, the V_A formula can be rewritten as:

$$\mathbf{V_A} = K(VCO_2 / PaCO_2)$$

where

K = factor (0.863) that converts CO_2 concentrations to pressure (mmHg)

■ 3. DIFFUSION OF GASES

Fick's First Law of Diffusion
The rate of diffusion across a membrane is quantitatively expressed by *Fick's first law of diffusion*:

$$V = \frac{D \times A \times (P_1 - P_2)}{\Delta X}$$

where

V = gas diffusion per unit time
D = diffusion constant for a particular gas
A = surface area of the membrane
$(P_1 - P_2)$ = partial pressure of the gas on either side of the membrane
ΔX = thickness of the membrane

Total Resistance Encountered By Oxygen
The *total resistance encountered by oxygen* ($1/D_L$) as it moves from the alveoli to combine with hemoglobin can be calculated by the following formula:

$$1/D_L = 1/D_M + 1/\theta Vc$$

where

$1/D_M$ = membrane resistance
$1/\theta Vc$ = chemical reaction resistance

Diffusing Capacity of a Gas
The *diffusing capacity of a gas* (D_L) can be calculated as:

$$D_L = \frac{V}{(P_A - P_C)} = mL / min / mmHg$$

where

V = uptake of gas per minute
$(P_A - P_C)$ = mmHg pressure difference of the gas

Carbon Monoxide Diffusion Capacity
For the *carbon monoxide diffusion capacity* (D_{LCO}), this generalized formula can be simplified to:

$$D_{LCO} = \frac{V CO}{P_A CO}$$

Because P_{CCO} remains near 0, it can usually be ignored in this equation.

■ 4. GAS TRANSPORT IN BLOOD

Oxygen Uptake
The difference between the inspired and expired fractional concentration of oxygen represents the *oxygen uptake* (VO_2):

$$\mathbf{VO_2} = (V_I \times F_IO_2) - (V_E \times F_EO_2)$$

where

V_I = volume of gas inhaled
F_IO_2 = fractional concentration of inspired oxygen
V_E = volume of gas exhaled
F_EO_2 = fractional concentration of expired oxygen

Oxygen in Solution in 100 mL of Blood
The amount of *oxygen in solution in 100 mL of blood* is calculated as (assuming a partial oxygen pressure of 70 mmHg):

$$(\mathbf{PO_2} / \mathbf{760}) \times \alpha O_2 = 70 / 760 \times 2.3 = 0.21 \text{ mL} / 100 \text{ mL}$$

P_{50}
The PaO$_2$ at which hemoglobin is 50 % saturated (P_{50}) can be calculated from the venous pH and arterial blood gases as:

$$\mathbf{P_{50}} = antilog\left(\frac{\text{Log } (1/k)}{n}\right) = \text{normal } 22 - 30 \text{ mmHg}$$

where

$$(\mathbf{1/k}) = (antilog[n \times \log \text{PaO}_{27.4}]) \times (100 - \text{SaO}_2 / \text{SaO}_2)$$

$$antilog[n \times \log \text{PaO}_{27.4}] = \log \text{PaO}_2 - 0.5(7.4 - \text{venous pH})$$

where

n = Hill constant = 2.7 for hemoglobin A

Fick Equation
The *Fick equation* for *oxygen consumption* (VO_2) is calculated as:

$$\textbf{VO}_2 = Q(CaO_2 - CvO_2)$$

where

Q = cardiac output (L/min)
CaO_2 = arterial oxygen content
CvO_2 = mixed venous oxygen content

CO_2 Production
The volume of carbon dioxide exhaled per unit time (*CO_2 production* or *VCO_2*) is calculated as:

$$\textbf{VCO}_2 = (V_E \times F_E CO_2) - (V_I \times F_I CO_2)$$

where

V_E = volume of gas exhaled per unit time
$F_E CO_2$ = fractional concentration of carbon dioxide in the exhaled gas
V_I = volume of gas inhaled per unit time
$F_I CO_2$ = fractional concentration of inspired carbon dioxide

Since the inspired gas usually contains negligible amounts of carbon dioxide, another representation of this formula is:

$$\textbf{VCO}_2 = V_E \times F_E CO_2$$

Oxygen Extraction Ratio
Another useful parameter in the characterization of tissue oxygenation is the *oxygen extraction ratio* (*ERO_2*), which is calculated with the following formula:

$$\textbf{ERO}_2 = \frac{VO_2}{TO_2} = \frac{(CaO_2 - CvO_2)}{CaO_2}$$

where

TO_2 = systemic oxygen transport = $Q \times CaO_2$ mL O_2/min

■ 5. PULMONARY CIRCULATION

Mean Pulmonary Artery Pressure
The *mean pulmonary artery pressure* (PAP) can be calculated utilizing the following formula:

$$\textbf{PAP} = (PVR \times PBF) + PAOP$$

where

PVR = pulmonary vascular resistance
PBF = pulmonary blood flow (which typically equals the cardiac output)

Pulmonary Vascular Resistance
Reorganizing the above formula, the *pulmonary vascular resistance* (PVR) is then
calculated as:

$$\mathbf{PVR} = (\text{Mean PAP} - \text{PAOP}) / \text{CO}$$

where

PAOP = pulmonary artery occlusion pressure
CO = cardiac output

Transmural Pressure
The pressures that surround the vessels in the pulmonary circulation contribute to the
transmural pressure (P_{tm}) represented as:

$$\mathbf{P_{tm}} = P_{vas} - P_{is}$$

where

P_{vas} = vascular pressure
P_{is} = perivascular interstitial pressure

Pulmonary Blood Flow
When the left atrial pressure (P_{la}) is available, the *driving pressure* responsible for
producing *pulmonary blood flow* is then calculated as:

$$(\mathbf{P_{pa}} - \mathbf{P_{la}}) = Q \times R_{vas}$$

where

P_{pa} = mean pulmonary arterial pressure
P_{la} = mean left atrial pressure
Q = pulmonary blood flow
R_{vas} = pulmonary vascular resistance

Pulmonary Vascular Compliance
The *pulmonary vascular compliance* (C_{vas}) can be calculated utilizing the following
formula:

$$\mathbf{C_{vas}} = \Delta V_{vas} / \Delta P_{vas}$$

where

ΔV_{vas} = change in blood volume
ΔP_{vas} = change in vascular pressure

Blood Flow Zones
The *blood flow zones* in an idealized upright lung with normal pressure differences are depicted in Table 12.2:

Table 12.2 Pulmonary blood flow zones

Blood flow zones	Pressures
I	$P_{alv} > P_{pa} > P_{pv}$
II	$P_{pa} > P_{alv} > P_{pv}$
III	$P_{pa} > P_{pv} > P_{alv}$
IV	$P_{pa} > P_{pv} > P_{alv}$

P_{alv} = pressure surrounding the alveolar vessels, P_{pa} = mean pulmonary arterial pressure, and P_{pv} = mean venous (left atrial) pressure

■ 6. MECHANICS AND GAS FLOW

Transpulmonary Pressure
The pressure inside the lungs relative to the pressure outside is known as the *transpulmonary pressure* (TP) and is calculated as:

$$\text{TP} = P_{alv} - P_{pl}$$

where

P_{alv} = alveolar pressure
P_{pl} = pleural pressure

Static Compliance
The change in volume (ΔV) for a unit pressure (ΔP) under conditions of no flow is the *static compliance*:

$$\text{Static compliance } (C_S) = \frac{\Delta V}{\Delta P}$$

Clinically, this formula can be simplified into:

$$C_S = \frac{V_T}{\text{Plateau airway pressure} - (\text{PEEP} + \text{auto-PEEP})}$$

where

V_T = tidal volume

Normal C_s value is 100 mL/cmH$_2$O

Dynamic Compliance
The *dynamic compliance* (C_{dyn}) can be calculated utilizing the following formula:

$$\mathbf{C_{dyn}} = \frac{V_T}{\text{Peak airway pressure} - (\text{PEEP} + \text{autoPEEP})}$$

Normal C_{dyn} value is 100 mL/cmH$_2$O.

Specific Compliance
The specific compliance (C_{spec}) is calculated utilizing the following formula:

$$\mathbf{C_{spec}} = C_{stat} / \text{FRC}$$

Chest Wall Compliance
The *chest wall compliance* (C_W) can be calculated as:

$$\mathbf{C_W} = \frac{V_T}{\text{Airway pressure} - \text{Atmospheric pressure}}$$

Separate Lung Compliance
Another formula that can be used under special circumstances (i.e., lung transplantation) is the *separate lung compliance* (C_X) and is calculated as:

$$\mathbf{C_X} = \frac{V_T}{\text{Airway pressure} - \text{Intrapleural pressure}}$$

auto-PEEP
If the tidal volume, chest compliance, expiratory time, and expiratory resistance are known, the *auto-PEEP* (AP) can be calculated utilizing the formula:

$$\mathbf{AP} = \frac{V_T}{C} \times \frac{1}{(e^{t_e/[(R_x)C]} - 1)} - \text{PEEP}$$

where

V_T = tidal volume
t_e = expiratory time
R_x = expiratory resistance
C = chest compliance

Poiseuille Equation
The type of gas flow in the lung is *laminar flow* and is described mathematically by
the *Poiseuille equation*:

$$\Delta P = \frac{8\mu l V}{\pi r^4}$$

where

ΔP = hydrostatic pressure drop
V = gas flow
μ = gas viscosity
l = path length
r = radius of the tube

From this equation resistance ($R = \Delta P/V$) can be calculated:

$$R = \frac{8\mu l}{\pi r^4}$$

The Pressure Drop During Turbulent Flow
On the other hand, *the pressure drop during turbulent flow* can be calculated utilizing
the following formula:

$$\Delta P = \frac{l\mu^{1/4}\rho^{3/4}V^{3/4}}{r^{19/4}}$$

where

ΔP = pressure drop during turbulent flow
μ = viscosity
ρ = density
r = radius
V = volume

Reynolds Number
The *Reynolds number* (*Re*) is the ratio of the pressure loss due to density dependent
or inertial flow versus the pressure loss due to viscous flow. This number is used to
predict the nature of a particular flow and is calculated as:

$$Re = \frac{2\rho r V}{\mu A}$$

Airway Resistance

The *airway resistance* (R_{aw}) using body plethysmography can be calculated utilizing the following formula:

$$\mathbf{R}_{aw} = \frac{\Delta V_{box}}{V} \times \frac{P_{alv}}{\Delta V_{box}} = \frac{P_{alv}}{V}$$

where

ΔV_{box} = volume changes in the box
V = flow
P_{alv} = alveolar pressure

Work of the Respiratory System

The *work of the respiratory system* (W) can be calculated as:

$$\mathbf{W} = P \times V$$

where

P = pressure
V = volume

◼ 7. VENTILATION/PERFUSION

Dead Space

The physiological *dead space* can be calculated utilizing the classic *Bohr equation*:

$$\mathbf{V_D} / \mathbf{V_T} = \frac{P_A CO_2 - P_E CO_2}{P_A CO_2}$$

where

$P_A CO_2$ = partial pressure of carbon dioxide in the alveolar gas
$P_E CO_2$ = partial pressure of carbon dioxide in mixed expired gas

Enghoff Modification

The above formula with the *Enghoff modification* is used in clinical practice:

$$\mathbf{V_D} / \mathbf{V_T} = \frac{P_A CO_2 - P_E CO_2}{P_a CO_2} = 0.2 - 0.35 \text{ in healthy subjects}$$

Quantity of Blood Passing Through Pulmonary Right-to-Left Shunts

The quantity of blood passing through pulmonary right-to-left *shunts* (Q_s/Q) is calculated as:

$$\mathbf{Q_s} / \mathbf{Q} = \frac{Cc'O_2 - CaO_2}{Cc'O_2 - CvO_2}$$

where

$$\mathbf{Cc\,'O_2} = (Hb \times 1.38) + P_A O_2 \times \frac{\alpha}{760}$$

Therefore, the Q_s/Q formula can be rearranged as:

$$\mathbf{Q_s} / \mathbf{Q} = \frac{(P_A O_2 - PaO_2) \times 0.0031}{(P_A O_2 - PaO_2) \times 0.0031 + (CaO_2 - CvO_2)}$$

■ 8. ALVEOLAR GAS EQUATION

Alveolar Air Equation

The *alveolar air equation* is based firmly on Dalton's law but is expressed in terms that emphasize alveolar O_2 and CO_2:

$$\mathbf{P_A O_2} = (P_{ATM} - P_{H_2O})F_i O_2 - PCO_2 / R_Q$$

where

$P_A O_2$ = partial pressure of O_2 in the alveolus under present conditions
P_{ATM} = current, local atmospheric pressure
P_{H_2O} = vapor pressure of water at body temperature and 100 % relative humidity
$F_i O_2$ = fraction of inspired O_2
PCO_2 = partial pressure of CO_2 in arterial blood
R_Q = respiratory quotient

At *sea level*, this equation can be simplified to:

$$\mathbf{P_A O_2} = 150 - 1.25 \times PaCO_2$$

Arterial Oxygen Tension
The *arterial oxygen tension (PaO$_2$) corrected for age* is calculated as:

$$\textbf{PaO}_2 \textbf{ age-corrected} = 100 - 1/3 \text{ age (in years)}$$

Alveolar–Arterial Oxygen Gradient
The *alveolar–arterial oxygen gradient* is *age-corrected* according to the following formula:

$$\textbf{Age correction} = 2.5 + (0.25 \times [\text{age in years}])$$

■ 9. PULMONARY FLUID EXCHANGE

Pulmonary Capillary Pressure
The *pulmonary capillary pressure* (P_{pc}) can be calculated utilizing the following formula:

$$\mathbf{P_{pc}} = P_{la} + (r_v / r_t)(P_{pa} - P_{la})$$

where

P_{la} = left atrial pressure
r_v/r_t = total vascular resistance
$P_{pa} - P_{la}$ = pressure gradient across the pulmonary circulation

Osmotic Pressure of Plasma
The following equation can be used to approximate the colloid *osmotic pressure of plasma* (Π_p):

$$\mathbf{\Pi_p} = 2.1C_p + 0.16C_p^{\,2}$$

where

C_p = serum protein concentration

Concentration of Protein in the Tissues
The concentration of protein in the tissues (C_T) relative to plasma (C_p) can be calculated as:

$$\mathbf{C_T / C_p} = \frac{(1 - \theta_d)J_v}{J_v} + \frac{P_S(C_P - C_T)}{J_v C_P}$$

where

  θ_d = osmotic reflection coefficient (solute selectivity of the pulmonary capillary wall)
  C_P = protein concentration of plasma
  J_v = capillary filtration
  P_S = permeability coefficient times the surface area for exchange

Starling Relationship
The movement of fluid across the capillary can be represented utilizing the *Starling relationship*:

$$\mathbf{J_v} = \text{filtration pressure} - \text{absorption pressure}$$

$$\mathbf{J_v} = K_{fc}[(P_{pc} - P_T) - \theta_d(\Pi_P - \Pi_T)]$$

where

  K_{fc} = solvent permeability of the pulmonary capillary wall

Normal Pressures in the Pulmonary Capillary Endothelium
The *normal pressures in the pulmonary capillary endothelium* are depicted in Table 12.3:

Table 12.3 Normal capillary endothelium filtration pressures

Parameter	Normal value
P_{pc}	7 mmHg
P_T	–5 mmHg
Π_P	28 mmHg
Π_T	17 mmHg
K_{fc}	0.02 mL/min/100 g/mmHg
θ_d	1

P_{pc} = capillary pressure, P_T = interstitial hydrostatic fluid pressure, Π_P = plasma colloid-osmotic pressure, Π_T = tissue colloid-osmotic pressure, K_{fc} = solvent permeability of the pulmonary capillary wall, and θ_d = solute selectivity of the pulmonary capillary wall

■ 10. VENTILATOR WEANING

Some of the standard indices predicting weaning success are depicted in Table 12.4:

Table 12.4 Standard indices for weaning success

Index	Value suggesting success
Minute ventilation (V_E)	<10 L/min
Tidal volume (V_T)	5 mL/kg
Vital capacity (VC)	$2 \times V_T$
Maximal voluntary ventilation (M_{VV})	$2 \times V_E$

Rapid Shallow Breathing Index
Another commonly employed weaning index is the *rapid shallow breathing index* (RSBI) which is calculated as:

$$\mathbf{RSBI} = f / V_T$$

where

f = frequency (breaths/min)
V_T = tidal volume (L)

Successful weaning is usually accomplished if the RSBI is <105 breaths/min/L

CROP
The *CROP* (acronym for compliance, rate, oxygenation, and pressure) index is an integrative index and is calculated with the following formula:

$$\mathbf{CROP\ index} = (C_{dyn} \times P_{imax} \times [PaO_2 / P_AO_2]) / \text{rate}$$

where

C_{dyn} = dynamic compliance
P_{imax} = maximal inspiratory pressure

Weaning success occur if value is ≥13 mL/breath/min.

■ 11. ACID–BASE FORMULAS

The reader is encouraged to also refer to the formulas and facts depicted in Chap. 8.

pH
The hydrogen ion concentration expressed in terms of pH is calculated as:

$$\mathbf{pH} = -\log[H^+]$$

Henderson–Hasselbach Equation
Using the *Henderson–Hasselbach equation* the pH is then calculated as:

$$\mathbf{pH} = p\mathrm{K} + \log \frac{[\mathrm{HCO_3^-}]}{[\mathrm{CO_2}]}$$

This equation can be applied clinically by modifying the formula as follows:

$$\mathbf{pH} = 6.1 + \log \frac{[\mathrm{HCO_3^-}]}{0.03\ P\mathrm{CO_2}}$$

Acute Respiratory Acidosis or Alkalosis
For *acute respiratory acidosis or alkalosis* the pH appropriate for acute in $\mathrm{PaCO_2}$:

$$\mathbf{\Delta pH\ (from\ 7.40)} = \Delta\mathrm{PaCO_2}\ (\text{from } 40\ \text{mmHg}) \times 0.007$$

Acute Respiratory Alkalosis
The bicarbonate level appropriate for change in $\mathrm{PaCO_2}$ is calculated in *acute respiratory alkalosis*:

$$\mathbf{Fall\ in\ HCO_3^-}\ (\text{from } 24\ \text{mmol} / \mathrm{L}) = 1 \text{ to } 3\ (\Delta\mathrm{PaCO_2} / 10)$$

Chronic Respiratory Alkalosis
The bicarbonate level appropriate for change in $\mathrm{PaCO_2}$ is calculated in *chronic respiratory alkalosis*:

$$\mathbf{Fall\ in\ HCO_3^-}\ (\text{from } 24\ \text{mmol} / \mathrm{L}) = 2 \text{ to } 5\ (\Delta\mathrm{PaCO_2} / 10)$$

Acute Respiratory Acidosis
The bicarbonate level appropriate for change in $\mathrm{PaCO_2}$ is calculated in *acute respiratory acidosis*:

$$\mathbf{Rise\ in\ HCO_3^-} = (\Delta\mathrm{PaCO_2} / 10) \pm 3$$

Chronic Respiratory Acidosis
The bicarbonate level appropriate for change in $\mathrm{PaCO_2}$ is calculated in *chronic respiratory acidosis* as:

$$\mathbf{Rise\ in\ HCO_3^-} = (\Delta\mathrm{PaCO_2} \times 4) / 10 \pm 4$$

Metabolic Acidosis
The compensatory *change in PaCO$_2$* for the degree of *metabolic acidosis* as expressed by a drop in bicarbonate is calculated as:

$$\textbf{Drop in PaCO}_2 = 1 \text{ to } 1.5 \times \Delta HCO_3^-$$

Metabolic Alkalosis
The compensatory *change in PaCO$_2$* for the degree of *metabolic alkalosis* as expressed by a rise in bicarbonate is calculated as:

$$\mathbf{\Delta PaCO}_2 = 0.25 \text{ to } 1.0 \times \Delta HCO_3^- \text{ (from 24 mmol / L)}$$

Bicarbonate Deficit (BD) in Metabolic Acidosis
To calculate the *bicarbonate deficit (BD) in metabolic acidosis*, the following formula is commonly employed:

$$\textbf{BD} = 0.5 \times (\text{weight in kg}) \times \Delta HCO_3^- \text{ (from 24 mmol / L)}$$

If the *pH is less than 7.1*, the formula is modified to:

$$\textbf{BD} = 0.8 \times (\text{weight in kg}) \times \Delta HCO_3^- \text{ (from 24 mmol / L)}$$

Anion Gap
The *anion gap* (AG) is calculated as:

$$\textbf{AG} = ([Na^+] + [K^+]) - ([Cl^-] + [HCO_3^-])$$

$$\textbf{AG normal} = 8 - 12 \text{ mEq(mmoL) / L}$$

■ 12. OTHER FACTS, FORMULAS, INDEXES, AND SCALES

Hyperbaric Oxygen Therapy
The approximate alveolar *PO$_2$* at different atmospheres during *hyperbaric oxygen therapy* (HBO) is depicted in Table 12.5:

Table 12.5 Effects of hyperbaric oxygen therapy at different environmental pressures on the alveolar PO_2

Environmental pressure (atmospheres)	Environmental pressure (mmHg)	Alveolar PO_2 breathing air (21 % oxygen)
1	760	102
2	1,520	262
3	2,280	422
6	4,560	902

Medical Research Council Dyspnea Scale

The *Medical Research Council Dyspnea Scale* (MRRC) is used to classify different stages of dyspnea in patients as depicted in Table 12.6:

Table 12.6 The Modified Medical Research Council Dyspnea Scale

Modified research council Dyspnea scale	
0	Breathless only with strenuous exercise
1	Short of breath when hurrying on the level or walking up a slight hill
2	Slower than most people of the same age on the level walking at own pace on the level
3	Stop for breath after walking about 100 m or after a few minutes at own pace on the level
4	Too breathless to leave house or breathless when dressing

BODE Index

The *BODE Index* (**B**ody mass index, airflow **O**bstruction, Modified Medical Research Council **D**yspnea scale, and **E**xercise capacity) is used to calculate the predicted 3-year mortality rate. It is depicted in Table 12.7:

Table 12.7 The BODE index and interpretation

The BODE Index				
Points	0	1	2	3
FEV_1% pred	≥65	50 – 64	36 – 49	≤35
6MWD (m)	≥350	250 – 349	150 – 249	≤149
MMRC	0-1	2	3	4
BMI (kg/m^2)	≤21	≥21		

Score	Three year mortality rate (chronically known pulmonary patients) %	Three year mortality rate (after first admission due to pulmonary obstructive disease) %
1	17.9	7.9
2	20.8	9.5
3	24.1	11.5
4	27.7	13.7
5	27.7	13.7
6	31.7	16.3
7	49.7	30.7
8	63.6	45
9	71.8	55
10	75.5	60

Borg Scale CR10 Scale
The *Borg Scale CR10 Scale* is used to document exertion during a physical test. It is depicted in Table 12.8:

Table 12.8 The Borg CR10 scale

0	Nothing at all
0.5	Very, very slight
1	Very slight
2	Slight
3	Moderate
4	Somewhat severe
5	Severe
6–7	Very severe
8–9	Very, very severe (almost maximal)
10	Maximal

GOLD Chronic Obstructive Pulmonary Disease Classification
The *GOLD Chronic Obstructive Pulmonary Disease Classification* is used to stratify patients with COPD as depicted in Table 12.9:

Table 12.9 The GOLD COPD Classification

Stage I	Mild COPD	$FEV_1/FVC < 70$	$FEV_1 \geq 80$ % normal
Stage II	Moderate COPD	$FEV_1/FVC < 70$	FEV_1 50–79 % normal
Stage III	Severe COPD	$FEV_1/FVC < 70$	FEV_1 30–49 % normal
Stage IV	Very severe COPD	$FEV_1/FVC < 70$	$FEV_1 < 30$ % or 50 % normal with chronic respiratory failure present

Flight PaO$_2$ Estimation
In *Flight PaO$_2$ estimation* is used to calculate if compromised patients traveling will need in cabin oxygen. The formula is as follows:

$$\text{Est. } \textbf{PaO}_2 = 1.59 + 0.98 \times pO_2 + 0.0031 \times \text{alt} - 0.000061 \times pO_2$$
$$\times \text{alt} - 0.000065 \times pCO_2 \times \text{alt} + 0.000000092 \times \text{alt}$$

where

pO_2 = arterial pressure of oxygen
pCO_2 = arterial pressure of CO_2
alt = flight altitude

Use of in-flight supplemental oxygen is recommended when PaO_2 is under 50–55 mmHg.

Oxygen Index
The *Oxygen Index* (OI) is used to measure the fraction of inspired oxygen and its use in the body. It can be used to evaluate the response to changes in inspired oxygen as:

$$\mathbf{OI} = \frac{100 \times F_iO_2 \times MAP}{PaO_2}$$

where

F_iO_2 = fraction of inspired oxygen
MAP = mean arterial pressure
PaO_2 = arterial pressure of oxygen

Hypoxemia Severity Index
The *Hypoxemia Severity Index* is used to assess severity of hypoxemia. The formula is as follows:

$$\mathbf{PIF} = PaO_2 / F_iO_2$$

For acute lung injury PIF is 200–300 mmHg; for acute respiratory distress syndrome PIF is <200 mmHg.

PISA Model for Pulmonary Embolism
The *PISA Model for Pulmonary Embolism* is used to aid in assessing the probability of pulmonary embolism. It is depicted in Table 12.10:

Table 12.10 PISA model for pulmonary embolism probability

Predictors	Points assigned
PISA model for pulmonary embolism	
Demographic characteristics	
Age	Age in years
Male	+10
Comorbid illnesses	
Cancer	+30
Heart failure	+10
Chronic lung disease	+10
Clinical findings	
Pulse ≥ 110/min	+20
Systolic blood pressure <100 mmHg	+30
Respiratory rate ≥ 30/min	+20
Temperature <36 °C	+20
Altered mental status	+60
Arterial oxygen saturation <90 %	+20

Classification	Sum of points
Class I, very low risk	≤65
Class II, low risk	66–85
Class III, intermediate risk	86–105
Class IV, high risk	106–125
Class V, very high risk	>125

PREP Score

The *PREP Score* is used to stratify the initial risk of adverse outcomes in patients with pulmonary embolism. An echocardiogram is required (Table 12.11):

Table 12.11 The PREP score

PREP score		
Prognostic factor	Categories	Points
Altered mental status	No	0
	Yes	10
Cardiogenic shock on admission	No	0
	Yes	6
Cancer	No	0
	Yes	6
BNP (ng/L)	<100	0
	100–249	1
	250–499	2
	500–999	4
	≥1,000	8
Right ventricle/left ventricle ratio	0.2–0.49	0
	0.5–0.74	3
	0.75–1.00	5
	1–1.25	8
	≥1.25	11

The points are summed and the patient is categorized as follows:

Classification	Points
Class I, low risk	≤6
Class II, intermediate risk	7–17
Class III, high risk	≥18

Community Acquired Pneumonia Severity Index (PORT Score)
The *Community Acquired Pneumonia Severity Index* (*PORT Score*) is used to classify patients depending on their risk for death and other adverse outcomes (Table 12.12):

Table 12.12 The PORT score

PORT Score	
Characteristic	**Points**
Demographic factors	
Age	
Men	Age (years)
Women	Age – 10 (years)
Nursing home resident	+10
Coexisting illnesses	
Neoplastic disease	+30
Liver disease	+20
Congestive heart failure	+10
Cerebrovascular disease	+10
Renal disease	+10
Physical examination findings	
Altered mental status	+20
Respiratory rate ≥ 30/min	+20
Systolic blood pressure < 90 mmHg	+20
Temperature <35°C or ≥ 40°C	+15
Pulse ≥ 125 /min	+10
Laboratory and radiographic findings	
Arterial pH < 7.35	+30
Blood urea nitrogen ≥ 30 mg/dl	+20
Sodium < 130 mmol/l	+20
Glucose ≥ 250 mg/dl	+20
Hematocrit < 30%	+10
Partial pressure of arterial oxygen < 60 mmHg	+10
Pleural effusion	+10

Classification	*Sum of Points*	*Mortality Rate*
Class I (absence of predictors)		0.1
Class II	≤ 60	0.6
Class III	71 – 90	2.8
Class IV	91 – 130	8.2
Class V	> 130	29.2

Wells Score

The *Wells Score* for clinical probability of pulmonary embolism is widely used and is depicted in Table 12.13:

Table 12.13 Wells score for pulmonary embolism

Wells score	
Variable	*Points*
Predisposing factors	
Previous deep venous thrombosis (DVT) or pulmonary embolism (PE)	+1.5
Recent surgery or immobilization	+1.5
Cancer	+1
Symptoms	
Hemoptysis	+1
Clinical signs	
Heart rate >100	+1.5
Clinical signs of DVT	+3
Clinical judgment	
Alternate diagnosis less likely than PE	+3

	Sum of points
Clinical probability (3 levels)	
Low	0–1
Intermediate	2–6
High	≥7
Clinical probability (2 levels)	
PE unlikely	0–4
PE likely	>4

Light's Criteria
In pleural effusions the *Light's Criteria* is commonly used to determine if an effusion is likely exudative. It must have at least one of the following:

• Ratio of pleural fluid protein to serum protein >0.5
• Ratio of pleural fluid LDH and serum LDH is >0.6
• Pleural fluid LDH is >0.7 times the normal upper limit for the serum

13

Renal, Fluid, and Electrolyte Facts and Formulas

Fluid and electrolyte balance is a challenging area of acute and critical care. In addition, renal problems are common, and their management incorporates a number of useful formulas and facts.

■ 1. ACID–BASE EQUATIONS/FACTS

Henderson Equation
The normal relationship between bicarbonate (HCO_3^-), hydrogen ions (H^+), and carbon dioxide is expressed in the *Henderson equation*:

$$[\mathbf{H}^+] = 24 \times (PCO_2 / [HCO_3^-])$$

where

PCO_2 = partial pressure of carbon dioxide

Henderson–Hasselbalch Equation
This interaction can also be represented by the *Henderson–Hasselbalch equation*:

$$\mathbf{pH} = 6.10 + \log([HCO_3^-] / [0.03 \times PCO_2])$$

J. Varon and R.E. Fromm Jr., *Acute and Critical Care Formulas and Laboratory Values*, DOI 10.1007/978-1-4614-7510-1_13, © Springer Science+Business Media New York 2014

The mean response equations for simple acid–base disturbances are depicted in Table 13.1:

Table 13.1 Selected response equations for simple acid–base disturbances

Acid–base disturbance	Equation
Metabolic acidosis	$\Delta PaCO_2 \approx 1.2\ \Delta[HCO_3^-]$
Metabolic alkalosis	$\Delta PaCO_2 \approx 0.7\ \Delta[HCO_3^-]$
Respiratory acidosis	
Acute	$\Delta[HCO_3^-] \approx 0.1\ \Delta PaCO_2$
	$\Delta[H^+] \approx 0.75\ \Delta PaCO_2$
Chronic	$\Delta[HCO_3^-] \approx 0.3\ \Delta PaCO_2$
	$\Delta[H^+] \approx 0.3\ \Delta PaCO_2$
Respiratory alkalosis	
Acute	$\Delta[HCO_3^-] \approx 0.2\ \Delta PaCO_2$
	$\Delta[H^-] \approx 0.75\ \Delta PaCO_2$
Chronic	$\Delta[HCO_3^-] \approx 0.5\ \Delta PaCO_2$
	$\Delta[H^+] \approx 0.5\ \Delta PaCO_2$

Amount of NaHCO₃

The amount of *NaHCO₃ needed* to raise the serum $[HCO_3^-]$ can be calculated as:

$$\textbf{NaHCO}_3\ \textbf{required (mEq)} = \text{Body weight (kg)} \times 0.7 \times (\text{Desired } [HCO_3^-] - \text{Current } [HCO_3^-])$$

Base Deficit

Alternatively, the following formula can be utilized to calculate the *base deficit* in metabolic acidosis:

$$\textbf{HCO}_3^-\ \textbf{deficit} = (\text{desired } HCO_3 - \text{observed } HCO_3) \times 0.4\ (\text{body weight (kg)})$$

Chloride Deficit
The *chloride deficit* in the treatment of metabolic alkalosis can be calculated utilizing the following formula:

$$\text{Cl}^- \textbf{ Deficit (mEq)} = 0.5 \text{ (weight in kg)} (103 - \text{measured Cl}^-)$$

■ **2. RENAL FUNCTION FORMULAS**

Glomerular Filtration Rate
The *glomerular filtration rate* (GFR) can be approximated, adjusted to age based on the following formulas:

$$\textbf{Below 45 years}: \text{GFR} = 12.49 - 0.37 \text{ (age)}$$

$$\textbf{At or above 45 years}: \text{GFR} = 153 - 1.07 \text{ (age)}$$

Cockcroft and Gault
A formula derived by *Cockcroft and Gault* is commonly used to estimate *creatinine clearance*:

$$\textbf{Creatinine clearance (mL / min)} = \frac{\text{Body weight (kg)}}{\text{Serum creatinine (mg/dL)}} \times \frac{140 \times \text{age}}{72}$$

In women, the value obtained from this equation is multiplied by a factor of 0.85.

Lean Body Weight
This formula can also be adjusted for lean body weight (LBW) calculated from:

$$\textbf{LBW (male)} = 50 \text{ kg} + 2.3 \text{ kg / in.} > 5 \text{ ft}$$

$$\textbf{LBW (female)} = 45.5 \text{ kg} + 2.3 \text{ kg / in.} > 5 \text{ ft}$$

Creatinine Clearance
Alternatively, the creatinine clearance (C_{cr}) can be calculated as:

$$\mathbf{C_{cr}} = \frac{(U_{cr} \cdot V)}{P_{cr}}$$

where

U_{cr} = concentration of creatinine in a timed collection of urine
P_{cr} = concentration of creatinine in the plasma
V = urine flow rate (volume divided by period of collection)

Jelliffe's Formula
Another commonly employed formula to calculate the creatinine clearance is *Jelliffe's formula*:

$$\mathbf{C_{cr}} = \frac{98 - 0.8\,(\text{age} - 20)}{P_{cr}}$$

In this formula, age is rounded to nearest decade. In females, the above result is multiplied by a factor of 0.9.

Mawer's Formula
A more complicated and potentially more accurate way to calculate creatinine clearance is *Mawer's formula*:

$$\mathbf{C_{cr}}\ (\textbf{males}) = \frac{\text{LBW}\,[29.3 - (0.203 \times \text{age})[1 - (0.03 \times P_{cr})]]}{14.4\,(P_{cr})}$$

$$\mathbf{C_{cr}}\ (\textbf{females}) = \frac{\text{LBW}\,[25.3 - (0.174 \times \text{age})[1 - (0.03 \times P_{cr})]]}{14.4\,(P_{cr})}$$

Hull's Formula
Hull's formula for creatinine clearance is calculated as:

$$\mathbf{C_{cr}} = [(145 - \text{age}) / P_{cr}] - 3$$

In females, the result is multiplied by a factor of 0.85.

Creatinine Clearance
Ranges for *creatinine clearance* under selected conditions are depicted in Table 13.2:

Table 13.2 Creatinine clearance values under selected conditions

Condition	Value (mL/min)
Normal	>85
Mild renal failure	60–85
Moderate renal failure	30–59
Severe renal failure	<30

■ 3. SELECTED ELECTROLYTES

Transtubular Potassium Gradient
The *transtubular potassium gradient* (TTKG) allows one to estimate the potassium secretory response in the cortical collecting duct. This index corrects for water reabsorption in the cortical and medullary collecting ducts as:

$$\textbf{TTKG} = \text{Corrected urine K}^+ / \text{Serum K}^+$$

$$\textbf{Corrected urine K} = \frac{\text{Urine K}^+}{U_{osm} / P_{osm}}$$

The normal renal conservation of potassium is reflected by a TTKG 8–9. During hyperkalemia, TTKG should be >10, low levels during hyperkalemia <7 may reflect mineralocorticoid deficiency (especially if accompanied by hyponatremia and high urinary sodium).

Magnesium Retention
The percentage of *magnesium retention* (MR) can be calculated by the following formula:

$$\textbf{MR}\,(\%) = 1 - \frac{\text{Postinfusion 24 h Mg} - (\text{Preinfusion urine Mg / Cr ratio} - \text{Postinfusion urine Cr})}{\text{Total elemental magnesium infused}} \times 100$$

Fractional Tubular Reabsorption of Phosphate
The *fractional tubular reabsorption of phosphate* (TRP) allows for quantification of renal phosphate wasting and is calculated as:

$$\textbf{TRP} = 1 - (C_{PO_4} / C_{cr}) \times 100$$

Normal is 80–95 %

where

C_{PO_4} / C_{cr} = fractional excretion of phosphate

Fractional Excretion of HCO_3^-
In conditions such as proximal renal tubular acidosis, the *fractional excretion of HCO_3^- ($F_E HCO_3^-$)* can be calculated as:

$$\textbf{F}_E\textbf{HCO}_3^- = \frac{\text{Urine } [HCO_3^-] \,(\text{mEq} / L)}{\text{Serum } [HCO_3^-] \,(\text{mEq} / L)} \times \frac{\text{Serum creatinine } (\text{mg} / dL)}{\text{Urine creatinine } (\text{mg} / dL)} \times 100$$

Correction of Calcium
The *correction of calcium* based on the serum albumin/globulin levels is calculated as:

$$\% \textbf{ Ca bound} = 8(\text{albumin}) + 2(\text{globulin}) + 3$$

Another formula to correct *calcium based on the total protein* is:

$$\textbf{Corrected Ca} = \text{measured Ca} / (0.6 + (\text{total protein} / 8.5))$$

A quick bedside formula for calculation of the corrected calcium:

$$\textbf{Corrected Ca} = \text{Calcium} - \text{albumin} + 4$$

■ 4. OSMOLALITY FORMULAS

Serum Osmolality
To calculate the *serum osmolality* (Osm), the following formula is employed:

$$\textbf{Osm} = 2Na^+ + \text{BUN} \,(\text{mg} / dL) / 2.8 + \text{glucose} \,(\text{mg} / dL) / 18$$

Osmolar Gap
The *osmolar gap* (OG) is calculated as the difference between the measured osmolality and the calculated osmolality:

$$\mathbf{OG} = \text{Measured osmolality} - \text{Calculated osmolality}$$

Urine Osmolality
The approximate *urine osmolality* can be calculated from the formula:

$$\mathbf{mOsm} \sim (\text{Urine specific gravity} - 1) \times 40{,}000$$

■ 5. WATER BALANCE

Total Body Water
To estimate the amount of *total body water* (TBW), the following formula is frequently employed:

$$\mathbf{TBW} = \text{Body weight (kg)} \times 60\,\%$$

Water Deficit
The *water deficit* of a patient can be estimated by the following equation:

$$\mathbf{Water\ deficit} = 0.6 \times \text{Body weight in kg} \times (P_{Na}/140 - 1)$$

where

P_{Na} = plasma sodium concentration

Free Water Deficit
Alternatively, the *free water deficit* from the osmolality can be calculated as:

$$\mathbf{H_2O\ deficit\ (L)} = \text{Total body weight (kg)} \times 0.6 \left(1 - \frac{\text{normal osm}}{\text{observed osm}} \right)$$

Free Water Clearance
To calculate the *free water clearance* based on the osmolar clearance, the following formula can be utilized:

$$\textbf{Free water clearance} = \text{Urine volume} - \text{Osmolar clearance}$$

where the *osmolar clearance* is calculated as:

$$\textbf{Osmolar clearance} = \frac{\text{Urine osmolarity} \times \text{urine volume}}{\text{Plasma osmolality}}$$

Excess Water
The *excess water* (EW) of a patient is calculated as:

$$\textbf{EW} = \text{TBW} - [\text{Actual plasma Na} / \text{Desired plasma Na}] \times \text{TBW}$$

■ 6. URINARY/RENAL INDICES

Urinary Indexes
The most common *urinary indexes* used in the differential diagnosis of acute renal failure are depicted in Table 13.3:

Table 13.3 Commonly used urinary indices in acute renal failure

Index	Prerenal	Acute tubular necrosis
Specific gravity	>1.020	<1.010
Urinary osmolality (mOsm/kg H_2O)	>500	<350
U_{osm}/P_{osm}	>1.3	<1.1
Urinary Na^+ (mEq/L)	<20	>40
U/P Cr	>40	<20
RFI	<1	>1
FENa (%)	<1	>1

Cr = creatinine, P = plasma, RFI = renal failure index, U = urine, and F_ENa = fractional excretion of sodium

Renal Failure Index
To calculate the *renal failure index* (RFI), the following formula is commonly employed:

$$\mathbf{RFI} = \frac{U_{Na}}{U / P_{Cr}}$$

Fractional Excretion of Sodium
The *fractional excretion of sodium* (F_ENa) is calculated as:

$$\mathbf{F_E Na} \ (\%) = \frac{\text{Quantity of Na}^+ \text{ excreted}}{\text{Quantity of Na}^+ \text{ filtered}} \times 100$$

or

$$\mathbf{F_E Na} \ (\%) = \frac{U / P_{Na^+} \times 100}{U / P_{Cr}}$$

or

$$\mathbf{F_E Na} \ (\%) = \frac{U_{Na} \times V}{P_{Na} \left(U_{Cr} \times V / P_{Cr} \right)} \times 100$$

or

$$\mathbf{F_E Na} \ (\%) = \frac{U_{Na} \times P_{Cr}}{P_{Na} \times U_{Cr}} \times 100$$

where

U_{Na} = urine sodium concentration
V = urine flow rate
P_{Na} = plasma sodium concentration
U_{Cr} = urine creatinine concentration
P_{Cr} = plasma creatinine concentration

■ 7. HEMODIALYSIS FORMULAS

The following are useful equations in the management of the chronic hemodialysis patient.

Protein Catabolic Rate

The *protein catabolic rate* (PCR) is calculated as:

$$\textbf{PCR (g / kg / day)} = 0.22 + \frac{0.036 \times \text{ID BUN} \times 24}{\text{ID interval}}$$

where

ID BUN = interdialytic rise in blood urea nitrogen (BUN) in mg/dL
ID = interval is the interdialytic interval in hours

Alternatively, if blood urea is measured the PCR can be calculated utilizing the following formula:

$$\textbf{PCR (g / kg / day)} = 0.22 + \frac{0.1 \times \text{ID urea} \times 24}{\text{ID interval}}$$

where

ID urea = interdialytic rise in blood urea in mmol/L

If the patient has a significant urine output, the contribution of the urinary urea excretion must be added to the PCR calculation and is calculated as:

$$\textbf{Urine contribution to PCR} = \frac{\text{Urine urea N (g)} \times 150}{\text{ID interval (h)} \times \text{Body weight (kg)}}$$

Alternatively, if urine urea is measured:

$$\textbf{Urine contribution to PCR} = \frac{\text{Urine urea (mmol)} \times 4.2}{\text{ID interval (h)} \times \text{Body weight (kg)}}$$

Percentage of Recirculation

To calculate the *percentage of recirculation* during hemodialysis, the following formula is utilized:

$$\textbf{\% Recirculation} = \frac{A2 - A1}{A2 - V} \times 100$$

where

A2 = blood urea or creatinine concentration in arterial blood line after blood pump is stopped
A1 = arterial line blood urea or creatinine concentration
V = venous line urea or creatinine concentration

Volume of Distribution of Urea
The *volume of distribution of urea* can be calculated as follows:

Males:

$$\mathbf{V} = 2.447 - 0.09516 \times A + 0.1074 \times H + 0.3362 \times W$$

Females:

$$\mathbf{V} = -2.097 + 0.1069 \times H + 0.2466 \times W$$

where

V = volume in liters
A = age in years
H = height in centimeters
W = weight in kilograms

Residual Renal Function
The calculation of *residual renal function* for dialysis three times per week:

$$\mathbf{GFR} = \frac{V \times U}{t \times (0.25\,U_1 + 0.75\,U_2)}$$

where

V = urine volume in interdialytic period
U = urine urea nitrogen or urea concentration
t = interdialytic period in minutes
U_1 = postdialysis BUN or blood urea on first dialysis of the week
U_2 = predialysis BUN or blood urea on second dialysis of the week

Percent Reduction of Urea
The *percent reduction of urea* (PRU) can be calculated utilizing the following formula:

$$\mathbf{PRU} = \frac{\text{Preurea} - \text{Posturea}}{\text{Preurea}} \times 100$$

Urea Reduction Ratio
The *urea reduction ratio* (URR) is calculated as:

$$\mathbf{URR} = 100 \times \left(1 - \frac{\text{Posturea}}{\text{Preurea}}\right)$$

■ 8. URINALYSIS

Please refer also to Chap. 17 for additional laboratory values. The most common *urinalysis* manifestations of renal diseases are depicted in Table 13.4:

Table 13.4 Urinalysis in different conditions

Condition	Findings
Prerenal failure	SG: >1.015 pH: <6 Prot: trace to 1+ Sed: sparse hyaline, fine granular cases or bland
Postrenal failure	SG: 1.010 pH: >6 Prot: trace to 1+ Hb: + Sed: RBCs, WBCs
Acute tubular necrosis (ATN)	"Muddy" brown urine SG: 1.010 pH: 6–7 Prot: trace to 1+ Blood: + Sed: RBCs, WBCs, RTE cells, RTE casts, pigmented casts
Glomerular diseases	SG: >1.020 pH: >6 Prot: 1 to 4+ Sed: RBCs, RBC casts, WBC, oval fat bodies, free fat droplets, fatty casts
Vascular diseases	SG: >1.020 if proglomerular pH: <6 Prot: trace to 2+ Sed: RBCs and RBC casts with glomerular involvement
Interstitial diseases	SG: 1.010 pH: –7 Prot: trace to 1+ Sed: WBCs, WBC casts, eosinophils, RBCs, RTE cells

RBC = red blood cells, RTE = renal tubular epithelial cells, WBC = white blood cells, SG = urine-specific gravity, Prot = protein, and Sed = urinary sediment

Some elements and substances can modify the color of urine in humans as depicted in Table 13.5:

Table 13.5 Urine color based on the presence of elements or substances

Elements/substances	Characteristic color
White blood cells Precipitated phosphates Chyle	Milky white
Bilirubin Chloroquine Sulfasalazine Nitrofurantoin Urobilin	Yellow/amber
Phenazopyridine Hemoglobin Myoglobin Red blood cells Phenothiazines Phenytoin Prophyrins Beets Red-colored candies	Brown/red
Melanin Phenol Methyldopa Metronidazole Quinine	Brown/black
Pseudomonas infection Amitriptyline Methylene blue Biliverdin Propofol	Blue/green

■ 9. OTHER FORMULAS/FACTS

Fractional Reabsorption of an AminoAcid
To determine whether a patient has aminoaciduria or not, the *fractional reabsorption of an amino acid* (FR_A) is determined utilizing the following formula:

$$\mathbf{FR_A} = 1 - k\left[\frac{[\text{Urine}]_A}{[\text{Plasma}]_A}\right] / \left[\frac{[\text{Urine}]_{Cr}}{[\text{Plasma}]_{Cr}}\right] \times 100\,\%$$

Urinary Excretion of Amino Acids
The normal *urinary excretion of amino acids* in patients older than 2 years is depicted in Table 13.6:

Table 13.6 Normal urinary excretion of selected amino acids.

Aminoacid	Normal excretion (mg/g of creatinine)
Cystine	18
Lysine	130
Arginine	16
Ornithine	22

Uric Acid Nephropathy
When acute renal failure (ARF) is due to *uric acid nephropathy* (*UAN*), the following equation is generally >1:

$$\textbf{Index} = \frac{\text{spot urine uric acid (mg / dL)}}{\text{spot urine creatinine (mg / dL)}} => 1.0$$

Urinary Anion Gap
Urinary Anion Gap helps find the source of the bicarbonate wasting process.

$$\textbf{AG}_U = Na_u + K_u - Cl_u$$

where

Na_u = urine sodium
K_u = urine potassium
Cl_u = urine chloride
$AG_U < 0$ indicates a gastrointestinal loss
$AG_U > 0$ distal or type IV RTA

Delta Gap
The *Delta Gap* is used to help differentiate between metabolic alkalosis and hyperchloremic acidosis.

$$\Delta\textbf{Gap} = Na - (Cl + HCO_3) + 0.25 \times (40 - Alb) - Gap_{nor} - 25 - HCO_3$$

14

Statistics and Epidemiology: Facts and Formulas

Although not commonly considered a clinical subject, statistics and epidemiology form the cornerstone of clinical practice. An understanding of statistical principles is necessary to comprehend the published literature and practice in a rational manner. The purpose of this chapter is to review some of the basic statistical principles and formulas. More in-depth discussion can be obtained in texts of biostatistics.

■ 1. MEASUREMENTS OF DISEASE FREQUENCY

Prevalence
Prevalence is the most frequently used measure of disease frequency and is defined as:

$$\text{Prevalence} = \frac{\text{Number of existing cases of a disease}}{\text{Total population at a given point in time}}$$

Incidence
Incidence quantifies the number of *new* cases that develop in a population at risk during a specific time interval:

$$\text{Cumulative incidence} = \frac{\text{Number of new cases of a disease during a given time period}}{\text{Total population at risk}}$$

J. Varon and R.E. Fromm Jr., *Acute and Critical Care Formulas and Laboratory Values*, DOI 10.1007/978-1-4614-7510-1_14, © Springer Science+Business Media New York 2014

Cumulative Incidence
Cumulative incidence (CI) reflects the probability that an individual develops a disease during a given time period. *Incidence density* (ID) allows one to account for varying periods of follow-up and is calculated as:

$$\mathbf{ID} = \frac{\text{New cases of the disease during a given period of time}}{\text{Total person-time of observation}}$$

Crude Mortality Rate
Special types of incidence and prevalence measures are reported. *Crude mortality rate* is an incidence measure:

$$\mathbf{Mortality\ rate} = \frac{\text{Number of deaths}}{\text{Total population}} \times 100,000$$

Case-Fatality Rate
Case-fatality rate is another incidence measure:

$$\mathbf{Case\ fatality\ rate} = \frac{\text{Number of deaths from the disease}}{\text{Number of cases of the disease}} \times 10^n$$

Attack Rate
Attack rate is also an incidence measure:

$$\mathbf{Attack\ rate} = \frac{\text{Number of new cases of the disease}}{\text{Total population at risk for a given time period}} \times 100$$

Secondary Attack Rate
Secondary attack rate (SAR) is also incidence measure:

$$\mathbf{SAR} = \frac{\#\,\text{new cases of the disease among contact of known cases}}{(\text{Population at beginning of the time period}) - (\text{primary cases})} \times 10^n$$

■ 2. LABORATORY TESTING

The performance of a laboratory test is commonly reported in terms of sensitivity and specificity defined as:

$$\mathbf{Sensitivity} = \frac{\text{True positives}}{\text{True positives} + \text{false negatives}}$$

$$\mathbf{Specificity} = \frac{\text{True negatives}}{\text{True negatives} + \text{false positives}}$$

Thus, *sensitivity* measures the number of people who truly have the disease who test positive. *Specificity* measures the number of people who do not have the disease who test negative.

These crude measurements of laboratory performance do not take into account the level at which a test is determined to be positive. *Receiver operator characteristics curves* (*ROC curves*) examine the performance of a test throughout its range of values. An area under the ROC curve of 1.0 is a perfect test, while a test that is no better than flipping a coin has an area under the ROC curve of 0.5.

Positive Predictive Value
As a clinician examining a positive test, we are most interested in determining whether a patient actually has disease. The *positive predictive value* (PPV) provides this probability:

$$\mathbf{PPV} = \frac{\text{True positives}}{\text{True positives} + \text{false positives}}$$

$$\mathbf{PPV} = \frac{\text{Prevalence x sensitivity}}{\text{Prevalence} \times \text{sensitivity} + (1 - \text{prevalence}) \times (1 - \text{specificity})}$$

Negative Predictive Value
Negative predictive value (NPV) describes the probability of a patient testing negative for the disease truly who does not have the disease:

$$\mathbf{NPV} = \frac{\text{True negatives}}{\text{True negatives} + \text{false negatives}}$$

$$\mathbf{NPV} = \frac{(1 - \text{prevalence}) \times \text{specificity}}{(1 - \text{prevalence}) \times \text{specificity} + \text{prevalence} \times (1 - \text{sensitivity})}$$

■ 3. DESCRIBING DATA

A large collection of data cannot be really appreciated by simple scrutiny. Summary or descriptive statistics help to succinctly describe the data. Two measures are usually employed: a measure of central tendency and a measure of dispersion.

Measures of Central Tendency
Measures of central tendency include mean, median, and mode. *Mean* is the common arithmetic average:

$$\mathbf{Mean} = \sum_{i=1}^{n} X_i \ / \ n$$

Median
Median is the middle value. The value such that one-half of the data points fall below and one-half falls above.

Mode
Mode is the most frequent occurring data point.

Measures of Dispersion
Measures of dispersion include the range, interquartile range, variance, and standard deviation.

$$\textbf{Range} = \text{Greatest value} - \text{Least value}$$

Interquartile Range
The *interquartile range* (IQR) is the range of the middle 50 % of the data.

$$\textbf{IQR} = U_{75} - L_{25}$$

where U_{75} is the upper 75th percentile and L_{25} is the lower 25th percentile.

Variance
Variance is the average of the squared distances between each of the values and the mean:

$$\textbf{Variance } (\mathbf{s^2}) = \frac{\sum (x - \bar{x})^2}{n-1}$$

Standard Deviation
Standard deviation is the square root of this value:

$$\textbf{Standard deviation } (\mathbf{s}) = \frac{\sqrt{\sum (x - \bar{x})^2}}{n-1}$$

■ 4. STATISTICAL TESTING

Hypothesis Testing
Hypothesis testing involves conducting a test of statistical significance, quantifying the degree to which random variability may account for the observed results. In performing hypothesis, testing two types of error can be made (see Table 14.1):

Table 14.1 Four possible outcomes of hypothesis testing

Conclusion of the test	Null hypothesis true	Alternative hypothesis true
Do not reject null hypothesis (not statistically significant)	Correct result: Is true, and we do not reject	Type II or beta error: Is true, but we do not reject
Reject null hypothesis (statistically significant)	Type I or alpha error: Is true, but we reject	Correct result: Is true and we reject

Type I Errors
Type I errors refer to a situation in which statistical significance is found when no difference actually exists. The probability of making a type I error is equal to the *p* values of a statistical test and is commonly represented by the Greek letter α. Traditionally, α levels of 0.05 are used for statistical significance. *Type II errors* refer to failure to declare a difference exists when there is a real difference between the study groups. The probability of making a type II error is represented by the Greek letter β. The *power* of a test is calculated as $1-\beta$ and is the probability of declaring a statistically significant difference if one truly exists.

■ 5. STATISTICAL METHODS

The following formulas and methods are the most frequently used test for biological data.

Chi-square Test
Chi-square test (χ^2) is used for discreet data such as counts. The general form of a chi-square test is:

$$\chi^2 = \sum \frac{(\text{Observed} - \text{expected})^2}{\text{Expected}}$$

Chi-square testing is commonly used in contingency tables (Table 14.2):

Table 14.2 Contingency table

	Diseased	Not diseased	Totals
Exposed	a	b	a+b
Not exposed	c	d	c+d
	a+c	b+d	a+b+c+d

where the expected frequencies for each cell of the contingency table is the product of the marginal totals divided by the grand total (see Table 14.3):

Table 14.3 Table of expected values

	Diseased	Not diseased
Exposed	$\dfrac{(a+c)(a+b)}{a+b+c+d}$	$\dfrac{(b+d)(a+b)}{a+b+c+d}$
Not exposed	$\dfrac{(a+c)(c+d)}{a+b+c+d}$	$\dfrac{(b+d)(c+d)}{a+b+c+d}$

Yates Correction
When the expected value of any particular cell is <5, the Yates correction is used. This is calculated as:

$$\chi^2 \text{ Yates corrected} = \sum \frac{(|\text{Observed} - \text{expected}| - 0.5)^2}{\text{Expected}}$$

Relative Risk
The data within a contingency table is commonly summarized in measures such as the relative risk. If we gather groups based on their exposure status, relative risk can be calculated as:

$$\text{Relative risk} = \frac{a/(a+b)}{c/(c+d)}$$

This figure represents the risk of becoming diseased if you are exposed ($a/a+b$) divided by the risk if you are not exposed ($c/c+d$), which is why it is called relative risk. If the relative risk is calculated at 4.0, then the risk of becoming diseased if you are exposed is four times that of people who are not exposed.

Odds Ratio
If we gather groups based on disease status, the odds ratio is calculated as an approximation to the relative risk:

$$\text{Odds ratio} = \frac{(a/b)}{(c/d)}$$

This measure is the ratio of the odds of getting disease if you are exposed and the odds of becoming diseased if you are not.

t-Test
Usually used in comparing means:

$$\text{2 sample independent } t\text{-test} = \frac{\bar{x}_1 - \bar{x}_2}{S_p\sqrt{\dfrac{1}{n_1} + \dfrac{1}{n_2}}}$$

with $(n_1 - 1) + (n_2 - 1)$ degrees of freedom
where

$$S_p = \frac{\sum(x_1 - \bar{x}_1)^2 + \sum(x_2 - \bar{x}_2)^2}{(n_1 - 1) + (n_2 - 1)}$$

$$\text{Paired } t\text{-test} = \frac{\text{Mean difference of the pairs}}{\text{SD}\left(\sqrt{\dfrac{1}{n}}\right)}$$

with $n - 1$ degrees of freedom.

Normal Approximation For Comparing Two Proportions
Normal approximation for comparing two proportions: A method for comparing whether two proportions are significantly different:

$$\mathbf{z} = \frac{P_1 - P_2}{\sqrt{\left(\dfrac{P_1 \times (1 - P_1)}{n_1}\right) + \left(\dfrac{P_2 \times (1 - P_2)}{n_2}\right)}}$$

Analysis of Variance
This method is commonly used to compare means across more than two categories.

Regression Techniques
Generally obtained via computer programs and can be used to predict a continuous variable from single or multiple regressors, which are either categorical, continuous, or both.

15

Toxicology Facts and Formulas

Toxic ingestions and intoxications are common reasons for emergency department presentation and admission to the intensive care unit. The following formulas, facts, and laboratory values may help the acute and critical care practitioner diagnose and manage these patients.

■ 1. BASIC FORMULAS

Therapeutic Index
The *therapeutic index* (TI) of a drug can be calculated as:

$$TI = \frac{LD50}{ED50}$$

where

LD50 = median lethal dose
ED50 = median effective dose

J. Varon and R.E. Fromm Jr., *Acute and Critical Care Formulas and Laboratory Values*, DOI 10.1007/978-1-4614-7510-1_15, © Springer Science+Business Media New York 2014

Margin of Safety

The *margin of safety* (MS) of a drug uses the ED99 for the desired effect and the LD1 for the undesired effect:

$$\mathbf{MS} = \frac{\text{LD1}}{\text{ED99}}$$

Apparent Volume of Distribution

The *apparent volume of distribution* (V_d) can be calculated by the following equation:

$$\mathbf{V_d} = \frac{\text{Dose}_{iv}}{C_0}$$

where

Dose_{iv} = intravenous dose

C_0 = extrapolated plasma concentration at time zero

The following formula is used to assess the *volume of the central compartment* (V_c):

$$\mathbf{V_c} = \frac{\text{Dose}_{iv}}{A + B}$$

where A and B represent disposition constants of a two-compartment model. In addition, the *peripheral compartment* (V_p) can be calculated as:

$$\mathbf{V_p} = \frac{\text{Dose}_{iv}}{B}$$

where B is derived from the elimination or equilibrium phase of a two-compartment model.

Total Body Clearance

The *total body clearance* (Cl) of a drug can be calculated as the sum of clearances by individual organs:

$$\mathbf{Cl} = Cl_r + Cl_h + Cl_i + \cdots$$

where

Cl_r = renal clearance

Cl_h = hepatic clearance

Cl_i = intestinal clearance

■ 2. OSMOLALITY FORMULAS

Serum Osmolality
To calculate *serum osmolality* the following formula is usually applied:

Calc. Osmolality (mOsm / kg) $= 2\text{Na} + \text{BUN} / 2.8 + \text{Glucose} / 18$

Osmolal Gap
The *osmolal gap (OG)* is useful in several intoxications and is calculated as:

OG $=$ Measured osmolality $-$ calculated osmolality

To calculate the contribution to measured osmolality of alcohols (also known as *osmol ratios*), the alcohol concentration (mg/dL) is divided by the numbers depicted in Table 15.1:

Table 15.1 Osmolal ratios of different alcohols

Ethanol	Ethylene glycol	Isopropanol	Methanol
4.6	6.2	6.0	3.2

■ 3. DIGITALIS INTOXICATION

In order to treat digitalis poisoning appropriately, it is important to assess the *digitalis body load*:

Body load (mg) $=$ (serum digoxin concentration) $\times$ (body weight in kg) $/ 100$

Dose of Digitalis Antibodies
The *dose of digitalis antibodies* (Digibind®) is determined by dividing the body load by 0.5 mg/vial:

Dose (number of vials) $=$ Body load (mg) $/ 0.5$ (mg / vial)

■ 4. MISCELLANEOUS

Rumack–Matthew Nomogram
The *Rumack–Matthew nomogram* for acetaminophen poisoning is depicted in Fig. 15.1:

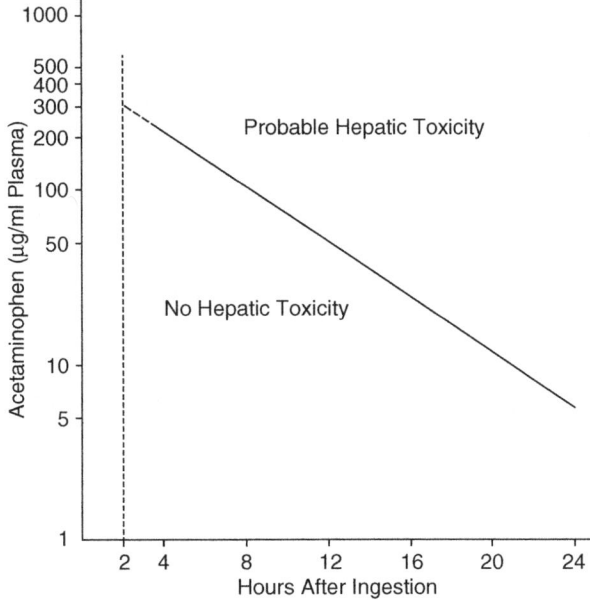

Fig. 15.1 Rumack–Matthew nomogram for acetaminophen poisoning

Done Nomogram

In acute salicylate poisoning, the *Done nomogram* is utilized to guide therapy and is depicted in Fig. 15.2:

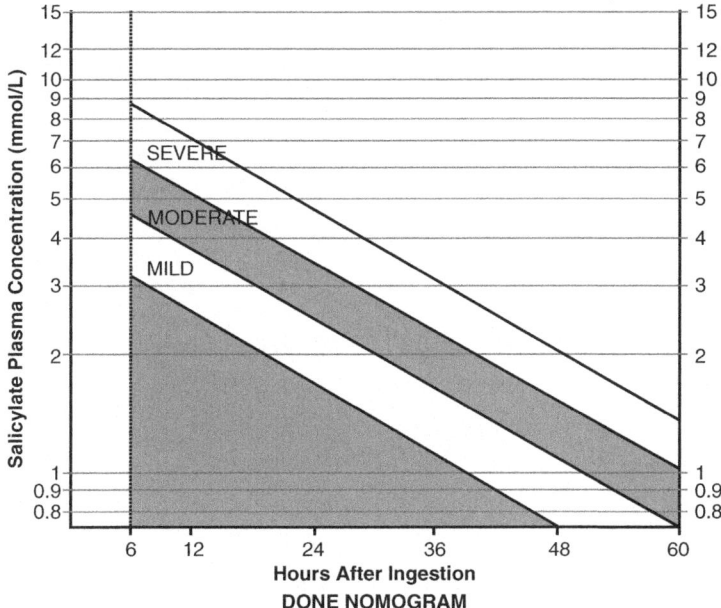

DONE NOMOGRAM

Fig. 15.2 Done nomogram for acute salicylate poisoning

Poison Control Centers
For any poisoning, it is recommended to notify the *poison control centers*. Telephone numbers for these centers are listed in Table 15.2:

Table 15.2 Telephone numbers for US regional poison control centers

State	City	800 number (in State only)	Telephone number
Alabama	Tuscaloosa	(800) 222 1222	
Alaska	Portland	(800) 222 1222	
Arizona	Tucson/Phoenix	(800) 222 1222	
Arkansas	Little Rock	(800) 222 1222	
California	San Francisco	(800) 222 1222	
Colorado	Denver	(800) 222 1222	
Connecticut	Farmington	(800) 222 1222	
Delaware	Philadelphia	(800) 222 1222	
District of Columbia	Washington, DC	(800) 222 1222	
Florida	Miami/Tampa	(800) 222 1222	
Georgia	Atlanta	(800) 222 1222	
Hawaii	Honolulu	(800) 222 1222	
Idaho	Denver, CO	(800) 222 1222	
Illinois	Chicago	(800) 222 1222	
Indiana	Indianapolis	(800) 222 1222	
Iowa	Sioux City	(800) 222 1222	
Kansas	Kansas City	(800) 222 1222	
Kentucky	Louisville	(800) 222 1222	
Louisiana	Monroe	(800) 222 1222	
Maine	Portland	(800) 222 1222	
Maryland	Baltimore	(800) 222 1222	
Massachusetts	Boston	(800) 222 1222	
Michigan	Detroit	(800) 222 1222	
Minnesota	Minneapolis	(800) 222 1222	

(continued)

Table 15.2 (continued)

State	City	800 number (in State only)	Telephone number
Mississippi	Jackson	(800) 222 1222	
Missouri	St. Louis	(800) 222 1222	
Montana	Denver, CO	(800) 222 1222	
Nebraska	Omaha	(800) 222 1222	
Nevada	Portland, OR	(800) 222 1222	
New Hampshire	Lebanon	(800) 222 1222	
New Jersey	Newark	(800) 222 1222	
New Mexico	Albuquerque	(800) 222 1222	
New York	New York	(800) 222 1222	
North Carolina	Charlotte	(800) 222 1222	
North Dakota	Minneapolis	(800) 222 1222	
Ohio	Columbus	(800) 222 1222	
Oklahoma	Oklahoma City	(800) 222 1222	
Oregon	Portland	(800) 222 1222	
Pennsylvania	Philadelphia	(800) 222 1222	
Rhode Island	Boston, MA	(800) 222 1222	
South Carolina	Columbia	(800) 222 1222	
South Dakota	Sioux Falls	(800) 222 1222	(605) 333-6638
Tennessee	Memphis	(800) 222 1222	
Houston	Dallas	(800) 222 1222	
Utah	Salt Lake City	(800) 222 1222	
Vermont	Portland, ME	(800) 222 1222	
Virginia	Richmond	(800) 222 1222	
Washington	Seattle	(800) 222 1222	
West Virginia	Charleston	(800) 222 1222	
Wisconsin	Milwaukee	(800) 222 1222	
Wyoming	Omaha, NE	(800) 222 1222	
Puerto Rico	San Juan		(787) 777-2770

16

Trauma Facts and Formulas

Trauma results in a number of emergency department presentations and intensive care unit admissions around the world and a number of formulas, scores, and indices are available for the assessment and management of these patients.

■ 1. HEMORRHAGE

In order to assess the intravascular volume resuscitation needed in a trauma patient, *normal blood volumes* according to age need to be known (see Table 16.1):

Severity of Hemorrhage
The *severity of hemorrhage* in a trauma patient can be classified as shown in Table 16.2:

Table 16.1 Normal blood volumes according to age

Normal blood volumes by age	
Newborn	85 mL/kg
Infant	80 mL/kg
Child	75 mL/kg
Adult	70 mL/kg

J. Varon and R.E. Fromm Jr., *Acute and Critical Care Formulas and Laboratory Values*, DOI 10.1007/978-1-4614-7510-1_16, © Springer Science+Business Media New York 2014

Table 16.2 Severity of hemorrhage classification trauma patients

Severity of hemorrhage	BP (mmHg)	Blood loss (mL)	Blood loss (%)	HR	Pulse pressure	RR	Urine output (mL/h)	CNS/mental status	Fluid replacement
Class I	Normal	>750	>15	<100	Normal or decreased	14–20	>30	Slightly anxious	Crystalloid
Class II	Normal	750–1,500	15–30	>100	Decreased	20–30	20–30	Mildly anxious	Crystalloid
Class III	Decreased	150–2,000	30–40	>120	Decreased	30–40	5–15	Anxious confused	Crystalloid and blood
Class IV	Decreased	>2,000	>40	>140	Decreased	>35	Negligible	Confused lethargic	Crystalloid and blood

BP blood pressure, *HR* heart rate, and *RR* respiratory rate

The following formula can be utilized to estimate how much whole blood or packed red blood cells (PRBCs) must be administered to change the hematocrit percentage to the desired amount in a trauma patient:

Transfusion required (mL) = Desired change in Hct × kg × factor

where

Hct = hematocrit
factor = varies with the volume of blood per body weight (adults and children >2 years, a factor of 1 will achieve a Hct of 70 % using PRBC and 1.75 to achieve a Hct of 40 % using whole blood)

■ 2. BURNS

Please refer also to Chap. 3.
There are several formulas that guide the initial fluid resuscitation after burn injuries. Below are the most common formulas used in clinical practice. In all these formulas, 50 % of calculated volume is given during the first 8 h, 25 % of calculated volume is given during the second 8 h, and 25 % of calculated volume is given during the third 8 h.
Fluids used for fluid management in major buns.

Parkland Formula
The *Parkland formula* can be calculated as:

< 24 h = Ringer's lactated (RL) solution 4 mL / kg / % burn
for adults and 3 mL / kg / % burn for children

RL solution is added for maintenance for children:

• 4 mL/kg/h for children 0–10 kg
• 40 mL/h + 2 mL/h for children of 10–20 kg
• 60 mL/h + 1 mL/kg/h for children of ≥20 kg

This formula recommends no colloid in the initial 24 h.

> 24 h = Colloids given as 20-60 % of calculated plasma volume

No crystalloids. Glucose in water is added in amounts required to maintain a urinary output of 0.5–1 mL/h in adults and 1 mL/h in children.
Modified formula:

< 24 h = RL 4 mL / kg / % burn (adults)

> 24 h = Begin colloid infusion of 5% albumin 0.3-1 mL / kg / % burn / 16 / h

Evans Formula
The *Evans formula* can be calculated as:

> **< 24 h** = Crystalloids 1 mL / kg / % burn plus colloids at 1 mL / kg /
> % burn plus 2,000 mL glucose in H_2O

> **> 24 h** = Crystalloids at 0.5 mL / kg / % burn, colloids at 0.5 mL / kg / % burn,
> and the same amount of glucose in water as in the first 24 h

Brooke Formula and the Modified Brooke Formula
The *Brooke formula* and the *modified Brooke formula* are calculated as:

> **< 24 h** = RL solution 1.5 mL / kg / % burn plus colloids 0.5 mL / kg /
> % burn plus 2,000 mL glucose in water

> **> 24 h** = RL 0.5 mL / kg / % burn, colloids 0.25 mL / kg / % burn,
> and the same amount of glucose in water as in the first 24 h

Modified formula = 2 mL Ringer's lactate/kg/% burn/24 h:

$$\text{< 24 h} = \text{No colloids}$$

RL solution 2 mL/kg/% burn in adults and 3 mL/kg/% burn in children.

> **> 24 h** = Colloids at 0.3-0.5 mL / kg / % burn and no crystalloids are given

Glucose in water is added in the amounts required to maintain good urinary output.

In addition to these formulas, the evaporative water losses in patients with burns need to be calculated and replaced.

Evaporative Water Loss
Evaporative water loss (EWL) is calculated as:

$$\text{EWL (mL / h)} = (25 + \% \text{ BSA burned}) \times \text{BSA}$$

■ 3. TRAUMA SCORING SYSTEMS

Out of the many used injury scoring systems, the abbreviated injury scale (AIS) is the most commonly used (see Table 16.3):

Table 16.3 The abbreviated injury scale

AIS score	Injury severity
1	Minor
2	Moderate
3	Serious
4	Severe
5	Critical
6	Unsurvivable

Trauma Score

The *trauma score* (TS) is another commonly utilized system and is depicted in Table 16.4:

Table 16.4 The trauma score

Variable	Measurements	Score
Respiratory rate (bpm)	10–24	4
	25–35	3
	> 35	2
	0–9	1
Respiratory effort	Normal	1
	Shallow, retractive	0
Systolic blood pressure (mm Hg)	>90	4
	70–90	3
	50–69	2
	<50	1
	No carotid pulse	0
Capillary refill	Normal	2
	Delayed	1
	Absent	0
Glasgow coma scale	14–15	5
	11–13	4
	8–10	3
	5–7	2
	3–4	1

Revised Trauma Score

The *revised trauma score* (RTS) eliminates the assessment of capillary refill and respiratory effort and is calculated as:

$$\textbf{RTS} = 0.9368\,\text{GCS} + 0.7326\,\text{SBP} + 0.2908\,\text{RR coded values} \\ \times \text{Revised score coefficient}$$

where

GCS = Glasgow coma scale
SBP = systolic blood pressure
RR = the respiratory rate

For children and infants, the *pediatric trauma score* is utilized (see Table 16.5):

Table 16.5 The pediatric trauma score

Variable	+2	+1	−1
Weight (kg)	>20	10–20	<10
Airway	Normal	Maintained	Non-maintained
Systolic BP (mm Hg)	> 90	50–90	<50
CNS function	Awake	Obtunded/loss of consciousness	Coma/decerebrate
Open wound	None	Minor	Major
Skeletal trauma	None	Closed	Open or multiple

■ 4. NEUROLOGICAL TRAUMA

AVPU Method

Within the primary survey, an early neurological trauma evaluation can be accomplished using the *AVPU method*:

A = *a*lert
V = responds to *v*erbal stimulation
P = responds to *p*ainful stimulation
U = *u*nresponsive

Glasgow Coma Scale

The *Glasgow coma scale* (Table 16.6) is another frequently utilized method of assessment of the neurological status of the trauma patient:

Table 16.6 Glasgow coma scale

Variable	Score
Eye opening	
Spontaneous	4
To verbal command	3
To pain	2
None	1
Best motor response	
Obeys verbal commands	6
Localizes painful stimuli	5
Flexion-withdrawal from painful stimuli	4
Decorticate (flexion) response to painful stimulation	3
Decerebrate (extension) response to painful stimulation	2
None	1
Best verbal response	
Oriented conversation	5
Disoriented conversation	4
Inappropriate words	3
Incomprehensible sounds	2
None	1

Cerebral Perfusion Pressure

In those patients with severe head injuries and intracranial pressure monitoring, *cerebral perfusion pressure* (CPP) is commonly utilized in management and is calculated as:

$$\textbf{CPP} = \text{MAP} - \text{ICP}$$

where

MAP = mean arterial blood pressure
ICP = intracranial pressure

Pressure–Volume Index

Another useful formula in neurological trauma is that of the calculation of the *pressure–volume index* (PVI), which is defined as the volume (in mL) necessary to raise the cerebrospinal fluid (CSF) pressure by a factor of 10:

$$\mathbf{PVI} = \frac{\Delta V}{\log 10(P_p / P_0)}$$

where

ΔV = volume change in the lateral ventricle using a ventricular cannula
P_0 = initial ICP
P_p = peak ICP

17

Common Laboratory Values

■ INTRODUCTION

The most common laboratory values used in the assessment of critically ill patients are presented in this chapter. They have been organized in alphabetical order and according to biologic source where (P) represents plasma, (B) blood, (S) serum, (U) urine, (CSF) cerebrospinal fluid, (RBCs) red blood cells, and (WBCs) white blood cells. These values are not intended to be definitive since normal ranges vary from hospital to hospital. Both traditional units and system international (SI) units are presented. The values may vary among different laboratories. We encourage the reader to consult their respective laboratory reference values.

α-1 Antitripsilin (S)
150–350 mg/dL (dual report) (*SI*: 1.5–3.5 g/L)

17-Ketogenic Steroids (as Dehydroepiandrosterone) (U)
Female: 7–12 mg/24 h (*SI*: 25–40 μmol/d)
Male: 9–17 mg/24 h (*SI*: 30–60 μmol/d)

17-Ketosteroids (as Dehydroepiandrosterone) (U)
Female: 6–17 mg/24 h (*SI*: 20–60 μmol/d)
Male: 6–20 mg/24 h (*SI*: 20–70 μmol/d)

Alanine Aminotransferase (ALT) (S)
0–35 (35 °C) Units/L (*SI*: 0–35 U/L)

Albumin (S)
4.0–6.0 g/dL (*SI*: 40–60 g/L)

J. Varon and R.E. Fromm Jr., *Acute and Critical Care Formulas and Laboratory Values*, DOI 10.1007/978-1-4614-7510-1_17, © Springer Science+Business Media New York 2014

Ammonia (P)

As ammonia (NH_3): 10–80 μg/dL (dual report) (*SI*: 5–50 μmol/L)
As ammonium (NH_4): 10–85 μg/dL (dual report) (*SI*: 5–50 μmol/L)
As nitrogen (N): 10–65 μg/dL (dual report) (*SI*: 5–50 μmol/L)

Amylase (S)

0–130 (37 °C) Units/L (*SI*: 0–130 U/L)
50–150 Somogyi units/dL (*SI*: 100–300 U/L)

Aspartate Aminotransferase (AST) (S)

0–35 (37 °C) Units/L (*SI*: 0–35 U/L)

Bilirubin (S)

Total: 0.1–1.0 mg/dL (dual report) (*SI*: 2–18 μmol/L)
Conjugated: 0–0.2 mg/dL (dual report) (*SI*: 0–4 μmol/L)

Calcium (S)

Male: 8.8–10.3 mg/dL (dual report) (*SI*: 2.20–2.58 mmol/L)
Female: <50 years 8.8–10.3 mg/dL (dual report) (*SI*: 2.20–2.58 mmol/L)

Calcium, Normal Diet (U)

<250 mg/24 h (*SI*: < 6.2 mmol/d)

Carbon Dioxide Content ($CO_2 + HCO_3$) (B,P,S)

22–28 mEq/L (*SI*: 22–28 mmol/L)

Chloride (S)

95–105 mEq/L (*SI*: 95–105 mmol/L)

Cholesterol (P)

<200 mg/dL (dual report) (*SI*: <5.20 mmol/L)

Cholesterol Esters, as a Fraction of Total Cholesterol (P)

60–75 % (*SI*: 0.60–0.75)

Complement C3 (S)

70–160 mg/dL (*SI*: 0.7–1.6 g/L)

Copper (S)

70–140 μg/dL (*SI*: 11.0–22.0 μmol/L)

Copper (U)

<40 μg/24 h (*SI*: <0.6 μmol/d)

Corticotropin (ACTH) (P)

20–100 pg/mL (*SI*: 4–22 pmol/L)

Creatine (U)

Male: 0–40 mg/24 h (*SI*: 0–300 μmol/d)
Female: 0–80 mg/24 h (*SI*: 0–600 μmol/d)

Creatine (S)

Male: 0.17–0.50 mg/dL (*SI*: 10–40 µmol/L)
Female: 0.35–0.93 mg/dL (*SI*: 30–70 µmol/L)

Creatinine (U)

Variable g/24 h (dual report) (*SI*: variable mmol/d)

Creatinine (S)

0.6–1.2 mg/dL (dual report) (*SI*: 50–110 µmol/L)

Creatine Kinase (CK) (S)

0–130 (37 °C) Units/L (*SI*: 0–130 U/L)

Creatine Kinase Isoenzymes, MB Fraction (S)

>5 % in myocardial infarction (*SI*: >0.05)

Creatinine Clearance (S, U)

75–125 mL/min (dual report) (*SI*: 1.24–2.08 mL/s)

Cystine (U)

10–100 mg/24 h (*SI*: 40–420 µmol/d)

Dehydroepiandrosterone (U)

Female: 0.2–1.8 mg/24 h (*SI*: 1–6 µmol/d)
Male: 0.2–2.0 mg/24 h (*SI*: 1–7 µmol/d)

Digoxin, Therapeutic (P)

0.5–2.2 ng/mL (dual report) (*SI*: 0.6–2.8 mmol/L)
0.5–2.2 µg/L (dual report) (*SI*: 0.6–2.8 mmol/L)

Erythrocyte Sedimentation Rate (B)

Female: 0–30 mm/h (*SI*: 0–30 mm/h)
Male: 0–20 mm/h (*SI*: 0–20 mm/h)

Estradiol, Male >18 years (S)

15–40 pg/mL (dual report) (*SI*: 55–150 pmol/L)

Ethyl Alcohol (P)

<100 mg/dL (*SI*: <22 mmol/L)

Etiocholanolone

Female: 0.8–4.0 mg/24 h (*SI*: 2–14 µmol/d)
Male: 1.4–5.0 mg/14 h (*SI*: 4–17 µmol/d)

Fibrinogen (P)

200–4,300 mg/dL (*SI*: 2.0–4.0 g/L)

Follicle-Stimulating Hormone (FSH) (P)

Female: 2.0–15.0 mIU/mL (*SI*: 2–15 IU/L)
Peak production: 20–50 mIU/mL (*SI*: 20–50 IU/L)

Male: 1.0–10.0 mIU/mL (*SI*: 1–10 IU/L)

Follicle-Stimulating Hormone (FSH) (U)

Follicular phase: 2–15 IU/24 h (*SI*: 2–15 IU/d)
Midcycle: 8–40 IU/24 h (SI: 8–40 IU/d)
Luteal phase: 2–10 IU/24 h (*SI*: 2–10 IU/d)
Menopausal women: 35–100 IU/24 h (*SI*: 35–100 IU/d)
Male: 2–15 IU/24 h (*SI*: 2–15 IU/d)

Gamma-Glutamyltransferase (GGT) (S)

0–30 (30 °C) Units/L (*SI*: 0–30 U/L)

Glucose (P)

70–110 mg/dL (dual report) (*SI*: 3.9–6.1 mmol/L)

Hematocrit (B)

Female: 36–46 % (*SI*: 0.33–0.43)
Male: 42–52 % (*SI*: 0.39–0.49)

Hemoglobin (B)

Male: 14.0–17.0 g/dL (*SI*: 140–180 g/L)
Female: 12.0–15.0 g/dL (*SI*: 115–155 g/L)

Hemoglobin (B)

Female: 12.0–15.0 g/dL (*SI*: 120–150 g/L)
Male: 14.0–17.0 g/dL (*SI*: 136–172 g/L)

Immunoglobulins (S)

IgG: 500–1,200 mg/dL (*SI*: 5.00–12.00 g/L)
IgA: 50–350 mg/dL (*SI*: 0.50–3.50 g/L)
IgM: 30–230 mg/dL (*SI*: 0.30–2.30 g/L)
IgD: <6 mg/dL (*SI*: <60 mg/L)
IgE:
0–3 years: 0.5–1.0 U/mL (*SI*: 1–24 μg/L)
3–80 years: 5–100 U/mL (*SI*: 12–240 μg/L)

Iron (S)

Male: 80–180 μg/dL (dual report) (*SI*: 14–32 μmol/L)
Female: 60–160 μg/dL (dual report) (*SI*: 11–29 μmol/L)

Iron-Binding Capacity (S)

250–460 μg/dL (dual report) (*SI*: 45–82 μmol/L)

Ketosteroid Fractions (U)

Androsterone

Female: 0.5–3.0 mg/24 h (*SI*: 1–10 μmol/d)
Male: 2.0–5.0 mg/24 h (*SI*: 7–17 μmol/d)

Lactate Dehydrogenase (S)

50–150 (37 °C) Units/L (*SI*: 50–150 U/L)

Lactate Dehydrogenase Isoenzymes (S)

LD_1: 15–40 % (*SI*: 0.15–0.40)
LD_2: 20–45 % (*SI*: 0.20–0.45)
LD_3: 15–30 % (*SI*: 0.15–0.30)
LD_4 and LD_5: 5–20 % (*SI*: 0.05–0.20)
LD_1: 10–60 Units/L (*SI*: 10–60 U/L)
LD_2: 20–70 Units/L (*SI*: 20–70 U/L)
LD_3: 10–45 Units/L (*SI*: 10–45 U/L)
LD_4 and LD_5: 5–30 Units/L (*SI*: 5–30 U/L)

Lead, Toxic (B)

>60 μg/dL (dual report) (*SI*: >2.90 μmol/L)

Lead, Toxic (U)

>80 μg/24 h (dual report) (*SI*: >0.40 μmol/d)

Lipids, Total (P)

400–850 mg/dL (dual report) (*SI*: 4.0–8.5 g/L)

Lipoproteins (P)

Low-density (LDL), as cholesterol: 50–190 mg/dL (dual report) (*SI*: 1.30–4.90 mmol/L)
High-density (HDL), as cholesterol:

Male: 30–70 mg/dL (dual report) (*SI*: 0.80–1.80 mmol/L)
Female: 30–90 mg/dL (dual report) (*SI*: 0.80–2.35 mmol/L)

Magnesium (S)

1.5–2.4 mg/dL (dual report) (*SI*: 0.80–1.20 mmol/L)

Mean Corpuscular Hemoglobin (B)

Mass concentration: 27–33 pg (*SI*: 27–33 pg)
Substance concentration (Hb[Fe]): 27–33 pg (*SI*: 1.68–2.05 fmol)

Mean corpuscular hemoglobin concentration (B)

Mass concentration: 33–37 g/dL (*SI*: 330–370 g/L)
Substance concentration (Hb[Fe]): 33–37 g/dL (*SI*: 20–23 mmol/L)

Mean Corpuscular Volume (B)

Erythrocyte volume: 76–100 cu μm (*SI*: 76–100 fL)

Phenytoin Therapeutic (P)

10–20 mg/L (*SI*: 40–80 μmol/L)

Phosphatase, Acid (prostatic) (P)

0–3 King–Armstrong Units/dL (*SI*: 0–5.5 U/L)

Phosphatase Alkaline (S)

30–120 Units/L (*SI*: 30–120 U/L)

Phosphate (as Phosphorus) (S)

2.5–5.0 mg/dL (dual report) (*SI*: 0.80–1.60 mmol/L)

Platelets (B)

200–500 × 10³/cu mm (*SI*: 200–500 × 10⁹/L)

Potassium (S)

3.5–5.0 mEq/L (*SI*: 3.5–5.0 mmol/L)

Progesterone (P)

Follicular phase: <2 ng/mL (*SI*: <6 nmol/L)
Luteal phase: 2–20 ng/mL (*SI*: 6–64 nmol/L)

Protein, Total (U)

<150 mg/24 h (*SI*: <0.15 g/d)

Protein, Total (S)

6–8 g/dL (*SI*: 60–80 g/L)

Protein Total (CSF)

<40 mg/dL (*SI*: <0.40 g/L)

Red Blood Cell Count (Erythrocytes) (B)

Female: 3.5–5.0 × 10⁶/cu mm (*SI*: 3.5–5.0 × 10¹²/L)
Male: 4.3–5.9 × 10⁶/cu mm (*SI*: 4.3–5.1 × 10¹²/L)

Red Blood Cell Count (CSF)
0/cu mm (*SI*: 0 × 10⁶/L)

Reticulocyte Count (Adult) (B)

10,000–75,000/cu mm (dual report) (*SI*: 10–75 × 10⁶/L)
Number fraction: 1–24 0/00 (No. per 1,000 erythrocytes) (*SI*: 1–24 × 10⁻³)
0.1–2.4 % (*SI*: 1–24 × 10⁻³)

Sodium (S)

136–145 mEq/L (*SI*: 136–145 mmol/L)

Sodium Ion (U)

Diet dependent mEq/24 h (*SI*: 5–25 mmol/d)

Steroids (U)

Hydroxycorticosteroids (as cortisol)

Female: 2–8 mg/24 h (*SI*: 5–25 μmol/d)
Male: 3–10 mg/24 h (*SI*: 10–30 μmol/d)

Testosterone (P)

Female: <0.6 ng/mL (dual report) (*SI*: <2.0 nmol/L)
Male: 4.0–8.0 ng/mL (dual report) (*SI*: 14.0–28.0 nmol/L)

Thyroxine (T_4) (S)

4–11 μg/dL (dual report) (*SI*: 51–142 nmol/L)

Thyroxine-Binding Globulin (TBG) (S)
12–28 µg/dL (dual report) (*SI*: 150–360 nmol/L)

Thyroxine Free (S)
0.8–2.8 ng/dL (dual report) (*SI*: 10–36 pmol/L)

Triiodothyronine (T$_3$) (S)
75–220 ng/dL (*SI*: 1.2–3.4 nmol/L)

Urate (as Uric Acid) (S)
2.0–7.0 mg/dL (*SI*: 120–140 µmol/L)

Urate (as Uric Acid) (U)
Diet dependent g/24 h (*SI*: diet dependent mmol/d)

Urea Nitrogen (S)
8–18 mg/dL (dual report) (*SI*: 3.0–6.5 mmol/L of urea)

Urea Nitrogen (U)
12–20 g/24 h (dual report) (*SI*: 430–700 mmol/d of urea)

Urobilinogen (U)
0–4.0 mg/24 h (*SI*: 0.0–6.8 µmol/d)

White Blood Cell Count (CSF)
0–5/cu mm (*SI*: $0–5 \times 10^6$/L)

White Blood Cell Count (B)
5,000–10,000/cu mm (*SI*: $3.2–9.8 \times 10^9$/L)

Zinc (S)
75–120 µg/dL (*SI*: 11.5–18.5 µmol/L)

Zinc (U)
150–1,200 µg/24 h (*SI*: 2.3–18.3 µmol/d)

Key Telephone Numbers

Department

J. Varon and R.E. Fromm Jr., *Acute and Critical Care Formulas and Laboratory Values*, DOI 10.1007/978-1-4614-7510-1, © Springer Science+Business Media New York 2014

Notes

_____

_____

_____

_____

_____

_____

_____

_____

_____

_____

_____

_____

_____

_____

Nursing Stations

_____

_____

_____

_____

_____

_____

Housing Staff

_____

_____

_____

_____

_____

_____

_____

_____

_____

_____

_____

_____

_____

J. Varon and R.E. Fromm Jr., *Acute and Critical Care Formulas and Laboratory Values*, DOI 10.1007/978-1-4614-7510-1, © Springer Science+Business Media New York 2014

Attending Staff

Other

Abbreviations

Abbreviated injury scale (AIS)

Acid phosphatase (S, P)

Actual reticulocyte count (ARC)

Acute renal failure (ARF)

Airway resistance (R_{aw})

Alanine aminotransferase (ALT)

Aldolase (S)

Alveolar pO_2 at sea level (P_AO_2)

Alveolar ventilation (V_A)

American Spinal Injury Association (ASIA)

Ammonia (P)

Anion gap (AG)

Antidiuretic hormone (ADH)

Apparent volume of distribution (V_d)

Arm muscle circumference (AMC)

Arterial blood O_2 content (CaO_2)

Arterial blood pressure (BP)

Arterial oxygen content (CaO_2)

Arterial oxygen saturation (SaO_2)

Arterial oxygen tension (PaO_2)

Arterial-jugular venous oxygen content difference ($AjvDO_2$)

J. Varon and R.E. Fromm Jr., *Acute and Critical Care Formulas and Laboratory Values*, DOI 10.1007/978-1-4614-7510-1,
© Springer Science+Business Media New York 2014

Arteriovenous oxygen difference ($avDO_2$)

Arteriovenous oxygen content difference [$avDO_2$]

Aspartate aminotransferase (AST)

Atrial pressure (P_{la})

Auto-PEEP (AP)

A–V oxygen content ($C(a-v)O_2$)

Blood urea nitrogen (BUN)

Basal energy expenditure (BEE)

Bethesda units (BU)

Bicarbonate (HCO_3)

Bicarbonate deficit (BD)

Body mass index (BMI)

Body surface area (BSA)

Calcium (S)

Calculate specimen concentration (C_u)

Carbon dioxide content ($CO_2 + HCO_3$)

Carbon monoxide diffusion capacity (D_{LCO})

Carboxyhemoglobin (B)

Cardiac index (CI)

Cardiac output (CO)

Catabolic index (CI)

Catabolic index (ID)

Celsius (°C)

Central venous pressure [CVP]

Cerebral blood flow (CQ)

Cerebral metabolic rate ($CMRO_2$)

Cerebral perfusion pressure (CPP)

Cerebrospinal fluid (CSF)

Chest wall compliance (C_W)

Chi-square test (χ^2)

Chloride (S,P)

Colloid osmotic pressure of plasma ($\mathbf{\Pi}_P$)

Community acquired pneumonia severity index (PORT score)

Concentration of protein in the tissues (C_T)

Coronary artery perfusion pressure (CPP)

Corrected reticulocyte count (CRC)

Cortisol (S,P)

Creatinine (S,P)

Creatinine height index (CHI)

Cumulative incidence (CI)

Daily protein requirements (PR)

Dead space volume (V_D)

Delivery date (DD)

Diabetes insipidus (DI)

Diastolic (PADP)

Diastolic blood pressure (DBP)

Dose of digitalis antibodies (Digibind®)

Dynamic compliance (C_{dyn})

Emergency departments (ED)

Endotracheal tube (ETT)

Evaporative water loss (EWL)

Excess water (EW)

Expiratory reserve volume (ERV)

Fahrenheit ($^{\circ}$F)

Fecal losses (FL)

Fetal peritoneal cavity (IPT volume)

Fibrinogen (P)

Follicle-stimulating hormone (FSH)

Fractional excretion of HCO_3^- ($FEHCO_3^-$)

Fractional excretion of sodium (F_ENa)

Fractional reabsorption of an amino acid (FR_A)

Fractional tubular reabsorption of phosphate (TRP)

Free thyroxine (fT_4)

Free triiodothyronine (fT_3)

Functional residual capacity (FRC)

Gamma-glutamyltransferase (GGT)

Glasgow Coma Scale (GSC)

Glomerular filtration rate (GFR)

Growth factor (GF)

Hyperbaric oxygen therapy (HBO)

Haptoglobin (S)

Hematocrit (B)

Humidity deficit (HD)

Harris–Benedict equation (HBE)

Ideal body weight (IBW)

Incidence density (ID)

Insensible losses (IL)

Inspiratory capacity (IC)

Inspiratory reserve volume (IRV)

Intensive care unit (ICU)

Internal diameter [I.D.]

Interquartile range (IQR)

Kelvin (K)

Lactate (B)

Lactate dehydrogenase (LDH) (S,P)

Lactate dehydrogenase Isoenzymes (S)

Last menstrual period (LMP)

Lead (B)

Lean body weight (LBW)

Left atrial pressure (LAP)

left ventricle (LV)

Left ventricular stroke work (LVSW)

Left ventricular stroke work index (LVSWI)

Lipase (S,P)

Local cortical cerebral blood flow (CBF)

Magnesium (RBC)

Magnesium retention (MR)

Manganese (S)

Margin of safety (MS)

Maximal voluntary ventilation (M_{VV})

Mean Arterial Pressure (MAP)

Mean corpuscular hemoglobin (MCH)

Mean corpuscular hemoglobin concentration (MCHC)

Mean corpuscular volume (MCV)

Mean pulmonary artery pressure (MPAP)

Median systolic blood pressure (SBP)

Medical Research Council Dyspnea Scale (MRRC)

Metabolic rate (MR)

Mid-upper arm muscle circumference (MUAMC)

Minimal plasma concentrations (C_{min})

Minute ventilation (V_E)

Mixed venous saturation (SvO_2)

Negative predictive value (NPV)

Nitrogen balance (NB)

Nonprotein caloric requirements (NCR)

Normal heart rate (HR)

Osmolar gap (OG)

Oxygen availability to neural tissue (CDO_2)

Oxygen capacity (B)

Oxygen consumption (VO_2)

Oxygen consumption index (VO_2I)

Oxygen delivery (DO_2)

Oxygen delivery index (DO_2I)

O_2 extraction (O_2 Ext)

Oxygen extraction index (O_2EI)

Oxygen extraction ratio (ERO_2)

Oxygen extraction ratio (OER)

Oxygen extraction ratio (O_2ER)

Oxygen index (OI)

Oxygen saturation [Venous] (B)

Oxygen uptake (VO_2)

Packed red blood cells (PRBC)

Partial pressure of alveolar CO_2 (P_ACO_2)

Partial pressure of arterial CO_2 ($PaCO_2$)

Partial pressure of arterial oxygen (PaO_2)

Partial thromboplastin time (P)

Percent reduction of urea (PRU)

Percentage of ideal body weight (%IBW)

Peripheral compartment (V_p)

Phosphorus, Inorganic (S,P)

Plasma (C_p)

Positive predictive value (PPV)

Potassium (RBC)

Potassium (S,P)

Pressure–volume index (PVI)

Probability of survival (POS)

Prognostic nutritional index (PNI)

Protein bound iodine (PBI)

Protein catabolic rate (PCR)

Prothrombin time (P)

Pulmonary artery occlusion pressure [PAOP]

Pulmonary artery pressure (PAP)

Pulmonary artery wedge pressure (PAWP)

Pulmonary capillary pressure (P_{pc})

Pulmonary right-to-left shunts (Q_s/Q)

Pulmonary vascular compliance (C_{vas})

Pulmonary vascular resistance (PVR)

Pulmonary vascular resistance index (PVRI)

Pulsatility index (PI)

Rapid shallow breathing index (RSBI)

Receiver operator characteristics curves (ROC curves)

Red blood cell count (CSF)

Red blood cells (RBC)

Relative humidity (RH)

Renal failure index (RFI)

Residual volume (RV)

Respiratory rate (RR)

Reticulocyte production index (RPI)

Revised trauma score (RTS)

Reynolds number (*Re*)

Right ventricular ejection fraction (RVEF)

Right ventricular end-diastolic volume (RVEDV)

Right ventricular end-systolic volume (RVESV)

Right ventricular stroke work (RVSW)

Right ventricular stroke work index (RVSWI)

Secondary attack rate (SRA)

Sedimentation rate (*B*)

Separate lung compliance (C_x)

Serum osmolality (Osm)

Sodium (S,P)

Specific compliance (C_{spec})

Steady state (C_{ss})

Stool osmolal gap (SOG)

Stool osmotic gap (SOG)

Stroke index (SI)

Stroke volume (SV)

Stroke volume index (SVI)

Systemic vascular resistance (SVR)

Systemic vascular resistance index (SVRI)

Systolic (PASP)

Systolic (SBP)

Therapeutic index (T_i)

Thrombin time (*P*)

Thymidine labeling index (TLI)

Thyroxine (T_4)

Thyroxine-binding globulin (TBG)

Tidal volume (VT)

Tidal volume (V_T)

Total body clearance (Cl)

Total body water (TBW)

Total daily energy (TDE)

Total lung capacity (TLC)

Total thyroxine (T_4)

Total triiodothyronine (T_3)

Transmural pressure (P_{tm})

Transpulmonary pressure (TP)

Transtubular potassium gradient (TTKG)

Trauma score (TS)

Triglyceride (S,P)

Triiodothyronine (T_3)

Urea Nitrogen (S,P)

urea reduction ratio (URR)

Uric acid (S,P)

uric acid nephropathy (UAN)

Urinary losses (UL)

urine urea nitrogen (UUN)

uterine venous blood flow (Sv)

Venous admixture (Q_{va}/Q_t)

Venous blood O_2 content (CvO_2)

venous oxygen content (CvO_2)

Vital capacity (VC)

Vital capacity (V_C)

Volume (B)

Volume (P)

Volume of distribution (V_D)

Volume of the central compartment (V_c)

Water (B,S,RBC)

White blood cell (WBC)

White blood cell count (CSF)

Work of the respiratory system (W)

Index

A

Abbreviated injury scale (AIS), 160–161
Acetaminophen, 152
Actual reticulocyte count (ARC), 46
Acute respiratory acidosis/alkalosis, 117
Alveolar air equation, 113
Alveolar–arterial oxygen gradient, 114
Alveolar ventilation, 104
American Spinal Injury Association (ASIA) scale, 67
Analysis of variance, 147
Anemias, 47–48
Anion gap (AG), 118
Antibiotics
    aminoglycoside clearance, 54
    levels of, 55
    pharmacokinetics, 53–54
Arm muscle circumference (AMC), 85
Arterial oxygen tension, 114
Attack rate, 142
AVPU method, 161

B

Basal metabolic rate, 90
Bicarbonate deficit (BD), 118
Biostatistics
    attack rate, 142
    case-fatality rate, 142
    crude mortality rate, 142
    cumulative incidence, 142
    incidence, 141
    negative predictive value, 143
    positive predictive value, 143
    prevalence, 141
    secondary attack rate, 142
    sensitivity and specificity, 142–143
Blood flow zones, 109
BODE index, 119–120
Body mass index (BMI), 31, 74, 89
Body surface area (BSA), 76, 86
Body weight estimation, 89
Bowman's formula, 81
Brooke formula, 160

C

Carbon monoxide diffusion capacity, 105–106
Cardiac index, 3, 6
Cardiovascular system
    advanced cardiovascular life support algorithms, 13
    adult tachycardia, 16, 17
    atrial fibrillation, 17
    atrial flutter, 18
    post-cardiac arrest care, 15
    pulseless ventricular tachycardia, 14

Cardiovascular system (*cont.*)
   supraventricular tachycardia,
     19
   Torsades de pointes, 20
   ventricular fibrillation, 14, 22
   ventricular tachycardia, 21
  alveolar arterial O_2 difference, 6
  arteriovenous O_2 difference, 6
  cardiac index, 6
  cardiac output, 4
  electrocardiography, 11–12
  heart rate measurement, 3
  hemodynamic parameter, 5–6
  mean arterial pressure, 6
  mean pulmonary arterial
    pressure, 7
  NYHA classification, 23
  O_2 consumption index, 7
  O_2 extraction and PVRI, 8
  oxygenation parameters, 7
  pacemaker, 9, 10
  pressure, 1
  primary determinant of, 2
  principle and conversion factor,
    2–3
  pulmonary to systemic flow
    ratio, 8
  stroke volume and SVRI, 8
Case-fatality rate, 142
Catabolic index (CI), 31, 74,
   84–85, 90
Cerebral blood flow (CBF)
  cerebral circulation, 60–61
  CPP, 61
  Hagen–Poiseuille equation, 61
  local cortical, 61–62
  pressure–volume index, 61
  pulsatility index, 62
Cerebral perfusion pressure (CPP),
   61, 163
Cerebrospinal fluid (CSF)
  composition of, 58
  etiological agents, 60
  multiple sclerosis, 60
  oncology, 85
  pressures and volumes, 57–58

  unknown etiology, 59
  values of, 59
Child–Pugh classification, 42
Chi-square test, 145
Chronic respiratory acidosis/
   alkalosis, 117
Cole formula, 87
Community acquired pneumonia
   severity index, 124–125
Corrected reticulocyte count
   (CRC), 46
Corticosteroids, 25–26
CPP. *See* Cerebral perfusion pressure
   (CPP)
Creatinine clearance, 130, 131
Creatinine height index (CHI), 74
Critically ill patients, laboratory values
  blood
    carbon dioxide content, 166
    erythrocyte sedimentation
     rate, 167
    hematocrit, 168
    hemoglobin, 168
    lead, toxic, 169
    MCH, 169
    MCV, 169
    platelets, 170
    red blood cell count, 170
    reticulocyte count, 170
    white blood cell count, 171
  cerebrospinal fluid
    protein, total, 170
    red blood cell count, 170
    white blood cell count, 171
  plasma
    ammonia, 166
    carbon dioxide content, 166
    cholesterol and cholesterol
     esters, 166
    corticotropin, 166
    digoxin, therapeutic, 167
    ethyl alcohol, 167
    fibrinogen, 167
    follicle-stimulating
     hormone, 167
    glucose, 168

lipids, total, 169
lipoproteins, 169
phenytoin therapeutic, 169
phosphatase, acid, 169
progesterone, 170
testosterone, 167
serum
alanine aminotransferase, 165
albumin, 165
amylase, 166
α1-antitrypsin, 165
aspartate aminotransferase, 166
bilirubin, 166
calcium, 166
carbon dioxide content, 166
chloride, 166
complement C3, 166
copper, 166
creatine, 167
creatinine and creatinine
clearance, 167
estradiol, 167
gamma-glutamyltransferase,
168
immunoglobulins, 168
iron and iron-binding capacity,
168
lactate dehydrogenase,
168, 169
magnesium, 169
MB fraction, 166
phosphatase alkaline, 169
phosphate, 169
potassium, 170
protein, total, 170
sodium, 170
thyroxine-binding globulin,
170
triiodothyronine, 171
urate, 171
urea nitrogen, 171
zinc, 171
urine
androsterone, 168
calcium, normal diet, 166
copper, 166

creatine, 167
creatinine and creatinine
clearance, 167
cystine, 167
dehydroepiandrosterone, 167
etiocholanolone, 167
follicle-stimulating hormone,
168
ketosteroid fractions, 168
17-ketosteroids, 165
lead, toxic, 169
protein, total, 170
sodium ion, 170
steroids, 170
urate, 171
urea nitrogen, 171
urobilinogen, 171
zinc, 171
Crude mortality rate, 142
CSF. *See* Cerebrospinal fluid (CSF)
Cumulative incidence (CI), 142

D
Dead space ventilation, 104
Diabetes insipidus (DI), 26
Diabetes mellitus, 27–28
Diabetic ketoacidosis (DKA), 28
Diastolic blood pressure (DBP), 88
Diffusing capacity, 105
Done nomogram, 155

E
Endocrinology and metabolism
adrenal function, 25–26
calcium metabolism and disorder,
30
diabetes insipidus, 26
diabetes mellitus, 27–28
hypoglycemia, 29
nutrition, 31
sodium and osmolality, 27
thyroid function test, 29–30
Endotracheal tube (ETT), 87, 88
Enghoff modification, 112

Environmental factors
    altitude, 38
    burns, 38–39
    humidity, 34–35
    pressure, 35–37
    temperature, 33
Eosinophils, 50
Evans formula, 160
Evaporative water loss (EWL), 160
Exchange transfusion, 92

F
Fick's first law, 105
Fluid and electrolyte balance
    acid–base equations/facts, 127–129
    aminoacid
        fractional reabsorption, 139
        urinary excretion, 140
    delta gap, 140
    electrolytes, 131–132
    hemodialysis formulas, 135–137
    osmolality formulas, 132–133
    renal function, 129–131
    uric acid nephropathy, 140
    urinalysis, 138–139
    urinary anion gap, 140
    urinary/renal indices, 134–135
    water balance, 133–134
Fractional excretion of sodium
    (F_ENa), 135
Fractional reabsorption, 139
Fractional tubular reabsorption of
    phosphate (TRP), 132
Free water clearance, 134
Free water deficit, 133
Functional residual capacity (FRC),
    102–103

G
Gastrointestinal system
    hepatitis, 42–43
    intestinal transit, 41, 42
    liver, 42

stool formulas, 41
Glasgow coma scale (GSC), 63–64,
    161–163
Glomerular filtration rate (GFR), 96,
    129, 137

H
Harris–Benedict equation, 31
Hematologic parameters
    acquired inhibitor, 50
    anemias, 47–48
    eosinophils, 50
    hemolytic disorder, 48–50
    HEMORR$_2$HAGES score, 51–52
    microscopic cell counting, 51
    plasma volume, 51
    red blood cells, 45–46
    reticulocytes count, 46–47
    transferrin saturation, 51
Hemoglobin rapid correction, 92
Hemolysis, 47
Hemorrhage, 51, 59, 157–159
Henderson equation, 127
Henderson–Hasselbalch equation,
    117, 127
Hepatitis, 42–43
Hull's formula, 130
Humidity deficit (HD), 34–35
Hyperbaric oxygen therapy (HBO),
    118–119
Hyperchloremic acidosis, 140
Hyperglycemia, 27
Hypoglycemia, 29
Hyponatremia, 27
Hypothesis testing, 144
Hypoxemia severity index, 122

I
Ideal body weight (IBW), 76
Incidence density (ID), 142
Interquartile range (IQR), 144
Intraperitoneal fetal transfusion
    (IPT), 81

J
Jelliffe's formula, 130

L
Laplace's law, 2
Lean body weight (LBW), 129
Left ventricular stroke work index
(LVSWI), 3
Lethal dose, 149

M
Magnesium retention (MR), 131
Margin of safety (MS), 150
Mawer's formula, 130
MCH. *See* Mean corpuscular
hemoglobin (MCH)
MCV. *See* Mean corpuscular volume
(MCV)
Mean, 143
Mean arterial pressure, 1
Mean corpuscular hemoglobin
(MCH), 45, 169
Mean corpuscular volume (MCV),
45, 169
Mean pulmonary artery pressure
(MPAP), 107–108
Measures of central tendency, 143–144
Measures of dispersion, 144
Median, 143
Median systolic blood pressure
(SBP), 88
Medical Research Council Dyspnea
Scale (MRRC), 119
Meningitis, 59
Metabolic acidosis/alkalosis, 118
Minute ventilation, 103–104
Mosteller formula, 89
Myocardial infarction, 15

N
Naegele's rule, 81
Negative predictive value (NPV), 143

Neurological illness
brain metabolism, 62–63
cerebral blood flow, 60–62
cerebrospinal fluid
composition of, 58
etiological agents, 60
multiple sclerosis, 60
pressures and volumes, 57–58
unknown etiology, 59
values of, 59
miscellaneous
$ABCD^2$ score, 65
apnea test, 64–65
ASIA scale, 67
CHA_2DS_2-VASC score, 67–68
dermatome map, 65–66
Glasgow coma scale, 63–64
modified Rankin scale, 68–69
muscle strength scale, 63
Ramsay sedation scale, 69
New York Heart Association
Functional (NYHA), 23
Nitrogen balance (NB), 31
Non-ketotic hyperosmolar coma
(HNKC), 28
Normal heart rate (HR), 88
Nutrition
assessment
body mass index, 74
catabolic index, 74
creatinine height index, 74
Harris–Benedict equation, 75
index of undernutrition, 73
injury factor, 72
metabolic rate, 72
nitrogen balance, 74
probability of survival, 73
prognostic nutritional index,
73
protein and nonprotein caloric
requirement, 74
total daily energy, 71–72
body surface area, 76
fuel composition, 75
ideal body weight, 76

O

Obstetrics and gynecology
    Bowman's formula, 81
    delivery date, 81
    hemodynamics
        labor and delivery, 77–78
        third trimester of pregnancy, 79
        uterine oxygen consumption,
            79–80
    intraperitoneal fetal transfusion, 81
    placental transfer of drug, 81–82
    pulmonary, 80
    weight gain, 81
Odds ratio, 146
Ohm's law, 2, 60–61
Oncology
    body surface area, 86
    carcinomatous meningitis, 85
    growth factor, 83
    nutrition
        arm muscle circumference, 85
        catabolic index, 84–85
        nitrogen balance, 84
        percent weight change, 84
    pericardial tamponade, 86
    thymidine labeling index, 83
Osmolal gap (OG), 133, 151
Osmolality, 151
Osmolar clearance, 134
Oxygen extraction ratio (OER/
    ERO_2), 62, 107
Oxygen index (OI), 122
Oxygen saturation, 79–80
Oxygen uptake, 106

P

Parkland formula, 158
Pediatrics
    airways, 87–88
    cation requirements, 91
    fecal losses, 91
    glucose infusion in newborns, 92
    hematological formulas, 91–92
    hemodynamics, 88
    insensible losses, 91

intravenous cannulation, 89
laboratory values
    acid–base measurements (B), 93
    acid phosphatase (S, P), 93
    alanine aminotransferase
        (ALAT, ALT, SGPT) (S), 93
    aldolase (S), 93
    ammonia (P), 93
    amylase, 93
    aspartate aminotransferase
        (ASAT, AST, SGOT) (S), 93
    bicarbonate serum, 94
    bilirubin serum, 94
    bleeding time (simplate), 94
    blood volume, 94
    calcium (S), 94–95
    carbon dioxide total (S, P), 95
    carboxyhemoglobin (B), 95
    chloride (S, P), 95
    cholesterol, total (S, P), 95
    cortisol (S, P), 95
    creatine kinase serum, 96
    creatinine (S, P), 96
    fibrinogen (P), 96
    glomerular filtration rate, 96
    haptoglobin (S), 97
    hematocrit (B), 97
    lactate (B), 97
    lactate dehydrogenase (LDH)
        (S, P), 97
    lead (B), 97
    lipase (S, P), 97
    magnesium (RBC, S), 97
    manganese (S), 97
    methemoglobin and
        sulfhemoglobin, 98
    osmolality, 98
    oxygen capacity (B), 98
    oxygen saturation [venous]
        (B), 98
    partial thromboplastin time
        (P), 98
    phosphorus inorganic (S, P), 98
    potassium, 98, 99
    prothrombin time (P), 99
    sedimentation rate (B), 99

sodium (S, P), 99
thrombin time (P), 99
triglyceride (S, P), 99
urea nitrogen (S, P), 99
uric acid (S, P), 99
volume (B, P), 100
water (B, S, RBC), 100
nutrition, 89–90
stool osmotic gap, 92
urinary losses (UL), 91
water requirements, 90
Percent reduction of urea (PRU), 137
Plasma osmotic pressure, 114
Plethysmography, 103
Poiseuille's law, 2
Portal hypertension, 42
Positive predictive value (PPV), 143
Pressure per square inch (Psi), 36
Pressure–volume index (PVI), 61, 164
Prevalence, 141
Prognostic nutritional index (PNI), 73
Protein catabolic rate (PCR), 136
Pulmonary blood flow, 108
Pulmonary capillary pressure, 114
Pulmonary disorders
    acid–base formulas, 116–118
    alveolar gas equation, 113–114
    BODE index, 119–120
    Borg Scale CR10 Scale, 120–121
    community acquired pneumonia
        severity index, 124–125
    flight PaO$_2$ estimation, 121–122
    gas diffusion, 105–106
    gas flow
        airway resistance, 112
        auto-PEEP, 110
        chest wall compliance, 110
        dynamic compliance, 110
        poiseuille equation, 111
        pressure drop during turbulent
            flow, 111
        respiratory system work, 112
        reynolds number, 111
        separate lung compliance, 110
        specific compliance, 110
        static compliance, 109–110

    transpulmonary pressure, 109
    gas transport, 106–107
    GOLD COPD classification, 121
    hyperbaric oxygen therapy, 118–119
    hypoxemia severity index, 122
    lung volumes, 101–103
    MRRC, 119
    oxygen index, 122
    PISA model, 122–123
    PREP score, 123–124
    pulmonary circulation, 107–109
    pulmonary fluid exchange,
        114–115
    pulmonary ventilation, 103–105
    ventilation/perfusion, 112–113
    ventilator weaning, 116
    wells score, 125–126
Pulmonary vascular compliance,
    108–109
Pulmonary vascular resistance index
    (PVRI), 8
Pulsatility index (PI), 62
Pulse pressure variation, 8–9

R
Rapid shallow breathing index
    (RSBI), 116
Receiver operator characteristics
    (ROC) curves, 143
Relative humidity (RH), 34
Relative risk, 146
Renal failure index (RFI), 135
Required packed cell volume, 91
Residual renal function, 137
Reticulocyte production index
    (RPI), 47
Reticulocytes, 46–47
Revised trauma score (RTS), 161
Rumack–Matthew nomogram, 152

S
Secondary attack rate (SAR), 142
Sepsis
    antibiotics

Sepsis (*cont.*)
    aminoglycoside clearance, 54
    kinetics, 53–54
    levels of, 55
  atypical mycobacteria, 55
Serum osmolality, 132, 151
Standard deviation, 144
Statistics and epidemiology
  analysis of variance, 147
  Chi-square test, 145
  data describing, 143–144
  disease frequency measurements,
    141–142
  hypothesis testing, 144
  laboratory testing, 142–143
  normal approximation, 147
  odds ratio, 146
  regression techniques, 147
  relative risk, 146
  statistical testing, 144–145
  t-test, 146
  type I errors, 145
  Yates correction, 146
Stool osmotic gap, 92
Systemic vascular resistance index
    (SVRI), 8

T
Therapeutic index (TI), 149
Thymidine labeling index (TLI), 83
Tidal volume, 103
Total body clearance (Cl), 150
Total body water (TBW), 133
Total daily energy (TDE), 71–72
Toxicology
  apparent volume of distribution, 150
  digitalis intoxication, 151
  Done nomogram, 153
  margin of safety, 150
  osmolality formulas, 151
  poison control centers, 154–155
  Rumack–Matthew nomogram, 152
  therapeutic index, 149

total body clearance, 150
Transtubular potassium gradient
    (TTKG), 131
Trauma
  abbreviated injury scale, 160–161
  burns, 158–160
  hemorrhage, 157–159
  neurological trauma
    AVPU method, 161
    cerebral perfusion pressure,
      163
    Glasgow coma scale, 163
    pressure-volume index, 164
  revised trauma score, 161, 162
  trauma score, 161, 162
t-test, 146
Type I errors, 145

U
Umbilical artery catheterization, 89
Umbilical vein catheterization, 89
Urea reduction ratio (URR), 137
Uric acid nephropathy (UAN), 140
Urinalysis, 138–139
Urinary anion gap, 140
Urinary excretion, 140
Urinary indexes, 134
Urine osmolality, 133
Uterine oxygen consumption, 79

V
Variance, 144
Vascular capacitance, 2
Vascular distensibility, 3

W
Water deprivation test, 26

Y
Yates correction, 146

31

The manufacturer's authorised representative in the EU is Springer
Nature Customer Service Centre GmbH, Europaplatz 3, 69115 Heidelberg,
Germany. If you have any concerns regarding our products, please
contact ProductSafety@springernature.com

Printed and bound by CPI Group (UK) Ltd, Croydon, CR0 4YY
23/04/2026
02095594-0001